Stepping On

Stepping On

Building Confidence and Reducing Falls

A community-based
program for older people

3rd edition
LINDY CLEMSON AND MEGAN SWANN

This edition published 2019 by Sydney University Press
First published 2003 by the University of Sydney
Second edition published 2008 by Sydney University Press

© Lindy Clemson and Megan Swann, 3rd edition, 2019

© Sydney University Press 2019

Reproduction and communication for other purposes

Sydney University Press
Fisher Library F03, University of Sydney
New South Wales 2006 AUSTRALIA
Email: sup.info@sydney.edu.au
Web: sydneyuniversitypress.com.au

A catalogue record for this book is available from the National Library of Australia

ISBN 9781743326640 paperback
ISBN 9781743326657 epub
ISBN 9781743326695 kindle

Book design by Duncan Blachford, Typography Studio

Exercise illustrations by Elena Fombertaux

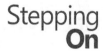

Stepping On is research based and scientifically proven to reduce falls.

The research for and development of this program was led by Professor Lindy Clemson, at the University of Sydney, Australia, and a report on a study of the program's effectiveness was accepted for peer-reviewed publication in the September 2004 issue of the *Journal of the American Geriatrics Society*.

That study was a randomised trial involving 310 people aged 70 and over who had experienced a fall in the previous 12 months, or who were concerned about falling. At the end of the 14-month study, those completing the Stepping On program had achieved an amazing 31 per cent reduction in falls. These results show that cognitive behavioural learning in a small-group environment can reduce falls.

Stepping On is a seven-week multifaceted group program supplemented by a follow-up visit or phone call to support and facilitate strategies adopted during the program. There is a booster session after three months, and we also recommend a six-month booster phone call.

The authors of this *Stepping On* manual are Professor Lindy Clemson and Megan Swann, with contributions from several other geriatric and fall-prevention experts. The third edition has been updated and revised following feedback from peers with academic and professional backgrounds.

Contents

3   Resources

Acknowledgements

Many thanks to all our participants – you taught us so much!

We acknowledge the contribution of our co-investigators in conducting the randomised trial of Stepping On: Professor Robert G. Cumming, Professor Hal Kendig, Robyn Twible, and our research assistant Kirsty Taylor. We particularly thank the late Robyn Twible for her passion for running group-based intervention and her lifelong commitment to community-based rehabilitation.

We also acknowledge Professor Jane Mahoney, University of Madison, Wisconsin, for her contribution to our manual and her commitment to dissemination of Stepping On in the USA.

Special thanks to Valerie Joy, Leichhardt Council, and the Balmain Leagues Club for getting us started with our first program and for providing support as we continued. We are extremely grateful to the Mercy Family Centre for a grant that helped us with program costs in those very early days.

We greatly appreciate the contributions made by Jenny Blennenhausen, Ewa Borkowski, Sandy Chech, Maureen Fitzgerald, Sarah Hilmer, Laverne Jaros, Valeree Lecey, Hylton Menz, Terry Shea, Esther Vance and finally Agata Mrva-Montoya from Sydney University Press.

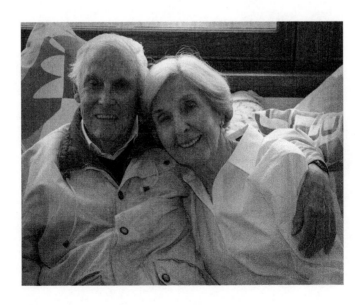

Introduction

The Stepping On program offers people a way of reducing falls and at the same time increasing self-confidence in situations where they are at risk of falling. The program incorporates a group setting plus individualised follow-up. It covers a range of issues, including falls and risks, strength and balance exercises, home fall hazards, safe footwear, vision and falls, safety in public places, community mobility, coping after a fall, and understanding how to initiate a medication review.

The *Stepping On* manual is designed for occupational therapists, physiotherapists, physical therapists, and other health professionals and health promotion staff who work with older people to prevent falls. Stepping On is a community-based fall prevention program. This program uses adult learning principles in a group setting over a seven-week period. It is about building self-confidence, making decisions, and behavioural change. It addresses the multifactorial nature of falls and draws on social cognitive theory to enable people to follow through with safety strategies. The program increases the older person's awareness of their own fall risk and subsequent behaviour change.

The manual describes how to plan, prepare, and run the program, and includes suggestions for evaluation.

Many older people have had a fall experience that has shaken their confidence and may have resulted in injury. They know that prevention of falls is vital to maintaining personal independence and engaging fully in their community. The program has been widely applied and received with enthusiasm.

....

'I have been referring older people at risk of falls to this program for years now. My patients love the common-sense practical approach and many of them continue to do the exercises for years after finishing the course. And I see the benefits in more confident older people who understand falls and how to reduce their risk of falling. It is a very empowering course for them. The biggest problem is that many of them want to do it again!'
– PROFESSOR SUSAN KURRLE, UNIVERSITY OF SYDNEY

....

....

'I regularly refer to Stepping On from our Osteoporotic Refracture Prevention Service. My patients not only benefit from the Stepping On program, they enjoy it! At a recent 12-month follow-up, a patient who had been a frequent faller proudly declared that she had done the program and hadn't had a single fall in over 12 months.'
– LILLIAS NAIRN, NORTH SHORE RYDE HEALTH SERVICE

....

'It's made me more aware, just so much more aware … of the buses … of my place … of making it brighter inside … of getting rid of leaves outside … of everything.'
– ROLEENA

....

'I've had some near falls, but you have a quicker recovery and your muscles don't collapse.'
– HERBERT

....

'It focuses on what elderly people can do, rather than what they can't. With an ageing population, the benefits of such a groundbreaking program are clear.'
– JOYCE

....

'We all have our abilities and disabilities. As we get older, the disabilities become more obvious. You lose some sight, some hearing, and maybe your balance is worse. But what *you* have done is focus on our abilities. No one else has done that.'
– NANCY

....

Important: All participants should have previously determined that they're medically fit for the moderate exercises taught in the program, and are doing so with the approval of their medical practitioner. They should notify instructors of any special needs or considerations beforehand. Instructors are not responsible for determining medical suitability for participating in this program.

AIMS OF THE PROGRAM

The Stepping On program:

- is designed to challenge participants to appraise their risks realistically, and to provide a forum within which they can gain knowledge about safety practices
- allows participants to determine risks and implement approaches that are personally relevant to them
- allows participants to explore options and barriers to putting safety strategies into practice
- makes it easier for the older person to have a sense of control of their risky behaviours and to explore different coping behaviours
- encourages the continued use of safety strategies in everyday life.

In short, Stepping On allows participants to identify hazards and risky behaviours, and then go on to problem-solve the issues; participants thus get a sense of ownership of the solutions that enhances follow-through. This process involves behaviour change.

To achieve these aims, the program is built on a sound conceptual basis. Decision-making theory[1] provides a basis for the Stepping On 'preventive framework'. There is a list of prompts that facilitators use throughout the program to facilitate the preventive process. The program draws on Bandura's[2] theory of self-efficacy, which describes techniques to enhance confidence in specific situations and make changes in our daily lives. Kwasnicka et al.[3] outline theoretical explanations for maintaining behavioural changes.

Stepping On includes specific practical strategies and resources that assist participants to self-regulate changes, and it taps into social and environmental influences to maintain self-selected actions and lifestyle changes.

Successful adult learning depends not only on expert health professional knowledge, but on an approach that actively builds on and uses the knowledge and experiences of the participant. Storytelling is one method used in the program to help achieve these aims.

It is clear that the program facilitator requires an understanding of group work, a commitment to working with older people, and a belief that falls can be prevented.

---

1   Janis & Mann, 1977.
2   Bandura, 1977; Bandura, 1997.
3   Kwasnicka, Dombrowski, et al., 2016.

WHO IS THIS PROGRAM FOR?

The group participants that we selected for our research and whom we recommend you recruit for the program are older people:

- who have had a fall in the past year or who have a fear of falling
- who are independent, with or without a walking stick
- who are cognitively intact
- who are living in the community
- who are able to speak conversational English or the language in which the group is facilitated.*

In the original research, people 70 years and over were recruited. Use your clinical judgement when recruiting younger people. People with Parkinson's disease or those with major neurological conditions affecting their mobility were not included and may need specialised and tailored evidence-based interventions.

HOW TO USE THIS MANUAL

The first chapter provides essential background reading to assist with understanding, running, and evaluating the program. This chapter also includes a section on marketing and recruitment, and the planning and resources required.

The program, as outlined in the main body of the manual, runs for seven weekly sessions, each of two hours' duration, including a coffee/tea break. These sessions are supplemented by a home visit by the program facilitator, to facilitate follow-through with preventive strategies and to assist with home adaptations as required. A letter is also sent out to the participant's doctor on the completion of the program. In our experience, the facilitator is an occupational therapist; however, this will vary for different organisations and contexts, depending on the availability and skills of staff. Some programs have provided a follow-up phone call instead of a home visit. Additional follow-up consists of a three-month booster session, and a six-month phone call to all participants.

---

* Translations of handouts are available in some additional languages. These can be downloaded from Sydney University Press: sydneyuniversitypress.com.au/stepping-on-2019

The manual begins by describing the steps needed to prepare and plan for the program. Each session is then outlined according to the following structure:

- objectives of the session
- checklist of resources required for the day
- outline of the session format
- detailed information to assist with running and presenting each segment ('topics').

Experts in the content areas are invited to facilitate segments within each session. Expert guest speakers are an essential component of this program. For example, an occupational therapist can lead the home fall hazard and other sections, the physical therapist (physiotherapist) can lead the exercise segment and answer relevant questions, and a medication expert (pharmacist) can be invited to discuss medications and falls. These segments are followed up with homework and revisited during other sessions.

The opportunity to become actively involved in reflection, discussion, questions, practice, and peer support is reinforced as the participants move through the decision-making process.

The topics provide more in-depth information about each content area. The handouts provided are designed to be useful to both the expert guest speaker and the group facilitator. Initially, our experts have not always had specific knowledge of how their content area relates to falls prevention.

The resources needed for the program (listed at the back of the manual) were current in 2019.

The handouts can be downloaded from Sydney University Press (sydney universitypress.com.au/stepping-on-2019) and reproduced freely with acknowledgement. They provide summaries of important points and are likely to be useful for reinforcing what is learned in program sessions. The facilitator distributes the handouts to participants after the discussion, unless the handout is specially needed for conducting an activity, in which case it is handed out during the session. Other community handouts can be placed on the resource table.

STEPPING ON PUBLICATIONS

The following is a list of research and other publications related to the
Stepping On programs.

Carande-Kulis, V., Stevens, J. A., Florence, C. S., Beattie, B. L., & Arias, I. (2015). A
cost-benefit analysis of three older adult fall prevention interventions. *Journal of
Safety Research, 52*, 65–70. doi: 10.1016/j.jsr.2014.12.007

Clemson, L., Cumming, R. G., Kendig, H., Swann, M., Heard, R., & Taylor, K. (2004).
The effectiveness of a community-based program for reducing the incidence of falls
among the elderly: a randomized trial. *Journal of the American Geriatrics Society,
52*(9), 1487–1494. doi: 10.1111/j.1532-5415.2004.52411.x

Liddle, J. L. M., Lovarini, M., Clemson, L. M., Jang, H. Y., Willis, K., Lord, S. R., & Sherrington, C. (2017). Men's perspectives on fall risk and fall prevention following
participation in a group-based programme conducted at Men's Sheds, Australia.
Health & Social Care in the Community, 25(3), 1118–1126. doi: 10.1111/hsc.12412

Mahoney, J. E. (2015). "Stepping On": stepping over the chasm from research to practice.
Frontiers in Public Health, 2, 148. doi: 10.3389/fpubh.2014.00148

Mahoney, J., Clemson, L., & Lovarini, M. (2015). Stepping On, a community-based fall
prevention program. In M. L. Malone, E. Capezuti, & R. M. Palmer (Eds), *Geriatrics
models of care: bringing 'best practice' to an aging America* (pp. 193–198). Cham,
Switzerland: Springer International Publishing.

Mahoney, J., Clemson, L., Schlotthauer, A., Mack, K., Shea, T., Gobel, V., & Cech, S. (2017).
Modified Delphi consensus to suggest key elements of Stepping On falls prevention program. *Frontiers in Public Health, 5*(4), 21. doi: 10.3389/fpubh.2017.00021

Mahoney, J. E., Gobel, V. L., Shea, T., Janczewski, J., Cech, S., & Clemson, L. (2016).
Improving fidelity of translation of the Stepping On falls prevention program through
root cause analysis. *Frontiers in Public Health, 4*, 251. doi: 10.3389/fpubh.2016.00251

Ory, M. G., Smith, M. L., Parker, E. M., Jiang, L., Chen, S., Wilson, A. D., Stevens, J. A.,
Ehrenreich, H., & Lee, R. (2014). Fall prevention in community settings: results from
implementing Stepping On in three states. *Frontiers in Public Health, 2*, 232. doi:
10.3389/fpubh.2014

Peterson, D. J., Christiansen, A. L., Guse, C. E., & Layde, P. M. (2015). Community
translation of fall prevention interventions: the methods and process of a randomized
trial. *Journal of Community Psychology, 43*(8), 1005–1018. doi: 10.1002/jcop.21728

Schlotthauer, A. E., Mahoney, J. E., Christiansen, A. L., Gobel, V. L., Layde, P., Lecey, V.,
… Clemson, L. (2017). Research on the translation and implementation of Stepping On
in three Wisconsin communities. *Frontiers in Public Health, 5*, 128. doi: 10.3389/
fpubh.2017.00128

Strommen, J., Brotherson, S., & Yang, Z. (2017). Older adult knowledge and behaviour
change in the Stepping On fall prevention program in a community setting. *Journal
of Human Sciences and Extension, 5*(3), 99–121.

Tiedmann, A., Sherrington, C., Lord, S., Purcell, K., & Clemson, L. (2019). Fall prevention
behaviour after participation in the Stepping On program: a pre-post study with
6-month follow-up. *Public Health Research & Practice*, in press.

BOOKS

Staying power is a companion book to *Stepping On* (available from Sydney
University Press, Amazon.com and Book Depository).

Clemson, L., & Swann-Williams, M. (2010). *Staying power: tips and tools to keep you on
your feet*. Sydney: Sydney University Press.

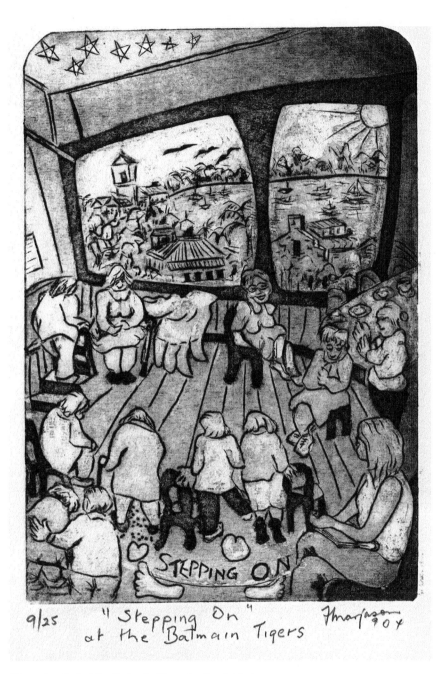

"Stepping On" at the Balmain Tigers by Frank Marjason.

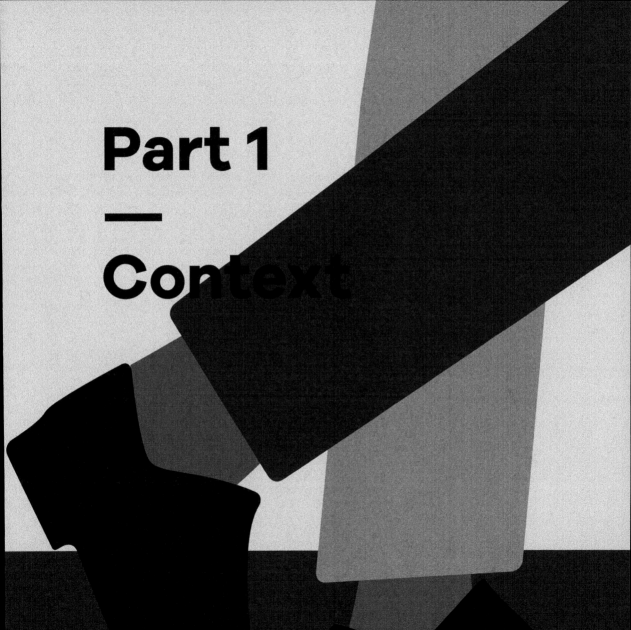

Part 1

—

Context

Background

This part provides background information essential for understanding the conceptual underpinning of the program and the group process.

The Stepping On program is designed to:

- use adult education principles to develop knowledge and skills for preventing falls, recognising that older adults have the capacity for learning and change
- increase awareness of falls risk and help people to be more informed about the factors contributing to their risk[1]
- enhance self-confidence in falls risk situations[2]
- utilise the decision-making process[3] to explore barriers and options and to develop skills in risk management
- boost follow-through with safety behaviours[4]
- target those behaviours that will have the most impact on reducing risk, and reinforce their application in the individual's home and community setting
- use a variety of learning strategies, including storytelling and the group process.

The program logit table provides an overview of the conceptual under-pinning and the program inputs (that is, the structure, content and components), and describes the impact and the outcome of the program.

This part also provides relevant ideas on recruitment of participants (based on our experience and that of others), and concludes with suggestions for evaluating the program.

---

1   Fischoff, 1989.
2   Bandura, 1995.
3   Janis & Mann, 1977.
4   Cole, Berger, & Garrity, 1988; Kwasnika, Dombrowski et al., 2016.

A program logit of the conceptual underpinning of Stepping On, Clemson & Swann, 2019.

CONCEPTUAL UNDERPINNING

- Adult learning principles
- Decision-making framework to prompt reflection and action
- Self-efficacy as a tool for change
- Reflective motivation
- Problem solving
- Support follow through with safety behaviours

PROGRAM STRUCTURE

- 7 two-hour weekly group sessions
- 10-12 participants per group
- Follow-up home visit
- 3-month booster session
- 6 month follow-up phone call

PARTICIPANTS

- Older people who fell in the past year or have a fear of falling
- Independent with or without a walking stick
- Cognitively intact
- Conversational English or language of the group

KEY CONTENT

- Balance and strength exercises
- Home hazard solutions
- Community safety
- Safe footwear
- Implementing medication reviews
- Low vision and falls
- What to do after a fall
- Vitamin D and calcium
- Public transport safety

KEY COMPONENTS

- Program leader facilitates meaningful engagement
- Peer engagement in solution generation, support and feedback
- Positive optimism and encouragement
- Use of story, prompts and cues
- Invited experts'/leader's key messages are clear and relevant
- Exercises and safety strategies linked to fall prevention
- Self-directed goal oriented appraisal
- Exercises reviewed and upgraded
- Outdoor mobility practice
- Weekly homework for action planning
- Review of homework and accomplishments

IMPACT

- Ability to analyse personal fall risk in different situations
- Understands why and how to challenge balance
- Sense of ownership of solutions
- Increased awareness of environment and identification of hazards
- Understands cues for self-monitoring quality of exercises
- Engages in balance and strength training at home and/or at a community class
- Safety strategies in place at home
- Mobility safety strategies used relevant to ability
- Talks to health professionals and doctor about medications

OUTCOME

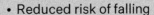

- Reduced risk of falling
- Maintains connection and engagement with community

The underpinning concepts: making decisions, learning and improving confidence

DECISION MAKING AS A PROCESS

The decision-making process is complex: it involves more than a brief two-phase process of giving advice and of that advice being accepted or otherwise. Commitment to action can waver or stop at any stage, and barriers to action can occur at any point. Janis and Mann[1] have identified five stages in decision making:

Stage 1 Appraising the challenge. In this stage, the person is exposed to an event or communication that conveys a threat or an opportunity. The response can be to ignore it, or to accept it and move on to the next stage.

Stage 2 Surveying the alternatives. Alternatives are considered and the person may actively seek advice and information about different ways of coping.

Stage 3 Weighing the alternatives. The possible advantages and disadvantages of each alternative are evaluated. What are the costs of the alternatives?

Stage 4 Deliberating about commitment. The person becomes increasingly committed to a course of action. This may involve speaking about the decision to others, thus demonstrating and reinforcing commitment.

Stage 5 Adhering despite negative feedback. The discouragement is dismissed and the person continues to implement the decision.

We have reframed the decision-making model in five simple questions (see below) to assist group facilitators in putting the model into practice. The questions are to be used as prompts in response to fall and safety stories in order to elicit helpful reflection and discussion.

---

1   Janis & Mann, 1977.

Such a schema recognises decision making as a process. There is evidence to support benefits from the application of this process in terms of their follow-through with environmental adaptations at home.[2] The model has also been applied to enhance follow-through with exercise programs. Hoyt and Janis[3] used a balance sheet procedure to interview women prior to an exercise class, asking them to consider the pros and cons of attending or not attending the activity class, and found this to be successful in increasing adherence. Using this kind of approach demonstrates a systematic way in which people can appraise risk, and assists them to move through the stages of decision making.

Preventive framework (for reflecting on fall stories)

1. What are the causes of falls, and what are the consequences?
2. How can you stop falls in the future?
3. How can you make this happen?
4. What are the barriers to you making this happen?
5. How can you keep this going? What are the benefits?

Adapting the framework to stories about safety strategies

1. Why did this work/not work and what are some other things that could work?
2. Which way works best for you?
3. How can you make this happen?
4. Are there any barriers to you making this happen?
5. How can you keep this going? What are the benefits?

The group facilitator can use this framework in all of the sessions, so we repeat it in each of the program chapters as a reminder.

The program initially concentrates on the participants' own appraisal of their risks before exploring risk-management strategies. Fischoff[4] demonstrated that risk-related information offered by experts is inadequate on its own. People need to be able to recognise and understand their risks themselves, and then move from risk appraisal to active problem-solving. In the initial sessions, the discussion centres on sharing fall stories, but as the program progresses, it becomes evident that the participants are actively engaged in making behavioural changes in daily routines. Group discussions then progress to stories about safety activities.

---

2   Clemson, Cusick, & Fozzard, 1998.
3   Hoyt & Janis, 1982.
4   Fischoff, 1989.

In the session after the one that covered safe footwear, a participant volunteered how she had been shopping for safe shoes that fitted the criteria she had learned ('fit, soles and support'). She had found a black pair in a particular local shop, but needed to find a blue pair as well. The ensuing conversation revolved around her achievement and where she could shop. She was evaluating her actions and reinforcing the learning of the essential elements of a safe shoe. This simple everyday story was one of many stories that reflected how valuable it can be for the participants to validate one another, and how storytelling can be part of committing ourselves to a particular course of action.

The approach used in the Stepping On program recognises the expertise of older people and the value of the safety strategies they already use, as well as the expertise of the health professional. Such an approach utilises the notion of exercising control[5] and choice[6] to support decision making. This can lead to the exploration of mastery experiences.

STORYTELLING – USING STORIES TO FACILITATE LEARNING AND DEVELOP CONFIDENCE

Storytelling and the use of stories can facilitate learning and the development of confidence in the area of falls prevention. We tell stories, we listen to stories, we encourage stories, and we prompt the participants to reflect on and use these stories in their decision making. The usefulness of storytelling can best be understood by looking into the literature on narrative. A story has a beginning, a middle, and an end. It is an account, unfolding in time and place, about an event or series of actions that is significant in some way for the narrator and for the audience.[7]

The event is recreated by the storytelling, and the narrative is about discovering the meaning that is attached to the story. Storytelling can be used to understand personal experiences and personal views. Through storytelling, our participants explore the negative events, describe and challenge their struggles to make changes, reaffirm the positive and what can be done differently in the future, and re-tell and recreate their stories with an evolving sense of personal control. Stories about a fall experience

---

5   Clemson, Cusick, & Fozzard, 1999.
6   Janis & Mann, 1977.
7   Polkinghorne, 1988; Turner, 1974.

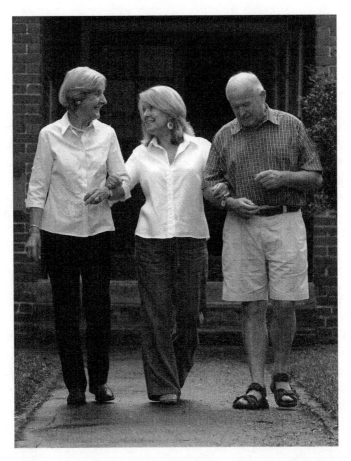

are important in understanding the motivation for change. It is the stories about solutions that can help mobilise us into action.[8]

Storytelling is a culturally familiar and cognitively effective teaching strategy.[9] Stories are more effective than facts or explanations alone in influencing thinking and behaviour. Learning occurs during the process of constructing and relating a story, as well as in the interpreting or making sense of that story.[10]

The facilitator and the participants can all make sense of the events and actions in their own way, and will have a range of viewpoints. The incident stories raise questions and give rise to a number of different interpretations. Alternative solutions can be suggested, and encouragement offered to the storyteller for coping with problems and change. Feelings of reduced self-efficacy in certain situations can reflect a self-identity linked to deterioration, fear of frailty, or frailty itself. The self-view of participants

8   Kendall-Taylor, 2017.
9   Fitzgerald, 2001; Kendall-Taylor, 2017.
10 Fitzgerald, 2001.

can be reframed as they feel stronger, become more confident in walking about, and become more informed about preventive strategies. The job of the facilitator is to assist with reframing, encouraging discussion about meaning, attitudes, and alternative solutions. This is done by guiding the participants through the preventive framework.

A story is rich in description. It gives the context of an experience, states the intentions and meanings that organise the experience in the storyteller's mind, and reveals the experience as a process.[11] Our stories are descriptions of everyday situations, yet encompass a rich variety of experience. Our stories tend to be short. However, because they can have meaning attached, they can be used to encourage reflective thinking and problem-solving.[12]

> Harry, a retired builder, is still climbing ladders to do his home maintenance. Does he believe this is unsafe? Is the way he does it unsafe? What are his alternatives? What are his intentions? What solutions can the group offer? If he is thinking of making changes to how he carries out his home maintenance, how can he put these changes into action? How important is it to his sense of self-worth that he continues to do the home maintenance? Is there a masculine identity aspect that needs to be understood in order to make sense of the choices made? Listening to Harry, and hearing the descriptive words he uses and the context of his story, can reveal his meaning. The real barriers can be revealed, reflected on, and tackled. As the story is told and interpreted, the group members can 'live' the experience and interpret it from their own perspective. Can we help Harry move forward, so he can open up to discussion and thinking about potential solutions within a positive and affirming environment?

We can make powerful and personal connections from a story based on our situation and perspective. When a story has personal meaning for us, our level of attention is heightened. Stories can engage us both cognitively and emotionally. And we remember stories much more than we remember numbers, graphs or PowerPoint presentations. **WE ALL LOVE STORIES!**

11　Denzin, 1994; Geertz, 1988.
12　Fitzgerald, 2001.

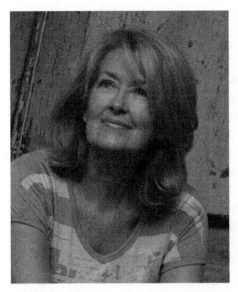

Stories should not remain stuck in a problem, but enable participants and the group to move towards affirming and solution-based discussions. The group can provide the opportunity and encouragement required for this.[13] The way the story is told is important, as is the interpretation. Some participants move easily into interpretation, and these people are valuable facilitators within the group. The stories and experiences are re-told in new ways as the discussion progresses. As participants learn and gain confidence in ways to prevent falls, they are able to put different interpretations on the event being described and can begin to reframe the stories.

Telling stories can make a person feel vulnerable, so it is important that the facilitator sets the scene from the first day, encouraging the telling of stories. By telling their own stories throughout the program, the facilitators demonstrate that they are prepared to be open and honest, thus developing trust and intimacy within the group. As trust is developed, the participants' stories will relate more significantly to personal experience.

'Marilyn and the cats' is a critical incident that we have developed from a story told by one of our participants. This critical incident could be used to stimulate discussion within the program, using one or two prompts to begin the conversation. For example:

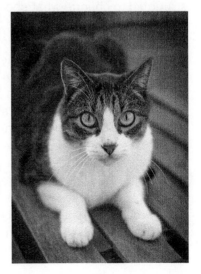

- What factors do you think may have contributed to Marilyn's fall?
- What could she do to be safer and feel more confident? How could she keep doing this?

13   Coleman, 1999.

Marilyn and the cats

Marilyn still lives with her daughter and granddaughter in the huge house in which she grew up in the inner city.

She said, 'It was just getting dark. I heard a "meow" in the backyard, so I went looking for my daughter's cats, as I was looking after them. She was away at the time. I could hear it: "Meow, meow". It was raining; I knew I shouldn't, but I went to see where they were and I walked out without my cane. I realised I could not see so well. My eyesight is not good. Here I am groping about in the dark, calling out the cat's name. I wouldn't normally go out at that time. I fell and really hurt my face.'

She added, 'And that's not all. I didn't learn. I did it again a few weeks later. "Meow, meow." And off to the backyard I go. But now I think, it's not worth having a fall. The cat's got nine lives, but I only have one, and I'm over 90 and I can't afford to lose it. The cat's okay; it came in for a meal!'

On reflecting and sharing this story Marilyn was able to affirm and implement a positive safe strategy.

Marilyn's narrative was also woven into the discourse of the group. She had struggled to change what she did naturally. She is used to looking after others and feels a strong sense of responsibility towards her daughter. She supports her daughter, a single mother, as much as she can. She is also a very intelligent and highly independent woman, still doing bookkeeping for a small accounting firm at the age of 91. Looking after others has always seemed to have much higher priority than investing time in her own personal wellbeing, but she is coming to terms with the idea that her wellbeing is important, and that there are things she can do to take better care of herself in her everyday actions. By the final group meeting, and on the subsequent home visit, she had changed her behaviours in some important ways to ensure her safety. She no longer goes looking for the cats in the dark, she takes her walking stick when she goes into the backyard, and she has slowed her pace. She has also installed a grab rail and sensor light at the back entrance to her home.

"STEPPING ON"

In our Falls Prevention Group
you learn a lot of things
New ways to get around
and we help your heart to sing.

There's going out, and moving round
and staying on your feet —
enjoying life in a larger field,
and there's new friends that you'll meet.

You'll learn to walk on gravel,
re-learn to climb up stairs —
to get in cars — and use a stick,
and climb out of a chair.

You learn to choose sun glasses
and how to check your visions,
and numbers of other little things,
to save you from collisions.

We learn new ways of moving round
with Megan Swann to show us,
and with new friends — it never ends —
even when the class is over.

And it doesn't finish there,
For those times that we hold dear,
It brings us all another chance
to live our life with cheer.

Yes, when our group is over,
they see us in our home —
an O.T. comes and checks us out —
that it's safe for us to roam.

So come along, and do the course,
we call it "STEPPING ON" —
You'll have a lot more happy days —
soon you'll find your fears have gone.

Yes, come along on your own —
with your partner — or man and wife,
For NOW you know, your time is prime —
get an extra lease of life.

(Frank M.)
'04

'Stepping On' by Frank Marjason.

The Stepping On stories are about falls, about ways of coping, about struggles to do things, but most of all about the need to move forward to changed attitudes, practical solutions, and shared achievements. They can be a cognitive analytic method of reflecting on what happened and why, and on what worked and how it worked. The facilitator's skill at telling stories, prompting stories, helping to develop the themes, and (sometimes) reframing the ideas that emanate from a story can help make these groups effective. Shared experiences become a valuable means of learning.

We use a variety of approaches. In the first session, the participants are asked to tell why they have come (a story in itself), and storytelling is encouraged at various other times. For instance, the weekly homework encourages participants to record their experiences, which can then be shared in the following session. In the final session, members reflect on what has changed in their lives as a result of their participation. Interpretation and reframing of stories occurs throughout the program, especially when discussing the incidents that are used as a stimulus for problem-solving in the 'Home fall hazards' session (see the critical incident above, or the story of Mrs Jardine or Mrs Mathews).

The simple questions of the adapted preventive framework mentioned before are prompts to elicit interpretation and decision making.

LEARNING, AND OLDER ADULTS AS LEARNERS

In our experience, people join Stepping On for a range of reasons: to prevent falls, to improve function or mobility, in response to pressure from others, to make new friends, to escape from mundane routine or depression, or for intellectual stimulation. Older people's major motivation for wanting to be part of the Stepping On program could be attributed to any one of these reasons, but they are all likely to gain a variety of positive experiences from the program.

There have been suggestions that older people learn best when the learning is self-paced. Self-paced learning allows enough time for learning, the benefits of breaks to reduce fatigue, and the opportunity to talk and receive optimistic and positive feedback. The use of visual aids and practical examples is helpful, and the tasks and material must be relevant. Building on previous experience and knowledge is also an effective technique for older learners. In fact, all of these approaches enhance learning for people of all ages and contribute to deeper-level learning.[14]

---

14   Hartley, 1998.

Working with older people requires the facilitator to ensure that the content is appropriate. Listening to and learning from participants, who will bring their own unique perspective, life stage and knowledge to the learning experience, is vital. The ability of older people to think analytically and creatively, as well as many of their practical skills, often match those of younger adults.[15]

Stereotyping by health professionals (and health professional students) of older adults and their capacity for learning and change can be a real barrier to the learning of older people. Societal views also influence the stereotyping of ageing by the older people themselves. Assumptions about and attitudes to their own learning can lead some older people to underestimate their own abilities and limit their potential. It is physical rather than cognitive factors that are more likely to differ for some older people. For example, apparent differences in listening ability and recall are more likely to be due to differences in learning style or in hearing, than cognitive ability.[16] Older people know when they are being spoken down to and not respected.

We have the capacity to learn throughout our life. We develop new neural connections and grow new nerve cells into our seventies, and very likely throughout the whole of life. Further, older people have a broad life experience to draw from. Older people have a great capacity for learning and change.

Like all learners, older people need to have an environment that encourages exploration outside their current knowledge, and opportunities for skill development. It is the responsibility of group facilitators to ensure that they and their co-presenters use good teaching practice. This means being positive and giving very clear instructions. It involves telling participants the aim of each segment or session. The intention of the program is to select important concepts and to offer effective ways of communicating them. Some concepts will require just a few minutes to convey, whereas others will take considerably longer. It is important to take enough time to explain the content clearly and to ensure that everyone understands; to encourage discussion; to be challenging; and to encourage participants to identify both the problems and their possible solutions.

A sense of ownership is highly conducive to learning. Some people will not ask questions in a group, but will give hints about their concerns as they arrive or during the coffee break, so it is important for group facilitators to listen for comments and asides.

---

15   Hartley, 1998.
16   Hartley, 1998; Schneider, Daneman, et al., 2000.

The learning experience can be enhanced by a range of visual, auditory and sensory aids to assist with learning. Different people learn in different ways. In addition, some people have special needs related to problems with hearing or vision. Group facilitators need to think laterally about opportunities for facilitating review, reflection and reinforcement.

Each segment or session should conclude with a summary of the important points covered, in addition to the homework recommended. Always ask at the beginning of each session: What three points can you remember from last week?

Deeper-level learning uses approaches that develop critical thinking and problem-solving. Reflection involves both thought and emotion, and occurs when people explore and evaluate their experiences – it can lead to new perspectives and new behaviours.[17]

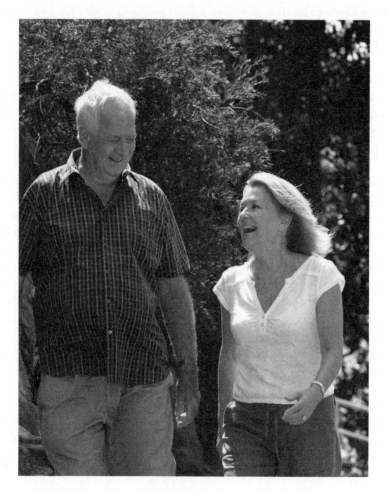

17   Boud, Keogh, & Walker, 1985; Egger, Spark, & Lawson, 1990.

THE PRINCIPLES OF ADULT EDUCATION

Group facilitators and guest speakers who use adult education principles:

- treat all members of the group as experts, and include all participants (not just the group facilitators and guest presenters)
- build on the experiences of the participants, allowing participants to bring their own perspectives and knowledge to the group
- share knowledge and have a personal interest in learning
- provide an atmosphere that encourages deep-level learning and reflection.

Education involves the development of both knowledge and skills, and the educational process is influenced by the attitudes, beliefs and values of the health professional, the older person, and the family, peer group, and community within which the older person lives.[18]

We consider the program to be a community-based intervention, and remind trainers of the influences of the participants' physical, social and cultural environments in shaping their learning and behaviours. We have deliberately chosen to run the program in community-based venues to help people situate and generalise newly acquired knowledge and skills into their everyday life.

The program aims to use a variety of learning approaches (to be explored further in this manual), such as the use of repetition, active engagement of participants in their learning (learning by doing), self-monitoring, and deeper-level reflection.

Older adult learners can have more difficulty concentrating if they have hearing or vision problems. Learning is often best achieved using a mix of auditory and visual materials (although some people are predominantly auditory learners or visual learners), so keep mixing up the learning aids, e.g. handouts/props/demonstrations.

Except for the 'Home Falls Hazards' we do not use slides. It is better to print a message on to posters or large cards, because this allows more interaction. Even the 'Home Falls Hazards' slides can be enlarged, laminated and made into large posters. They can then become props that can be passed around. This allows participants to engage with the pictures, identify hazards, and problem-solve, thus developing a sense of ownership that encourages follow-through.

---

18   Egger, Spark, & Lawson, 1990.

We do not use slides because they tend to lock a talk into a course that disregards any input other than the speaker's own ideas. They tend to restrict participant engagement and are a poor tool for reflection. We aim to encourage spontaneous questions and the participants' ideas. The Stepping On facilitator needs to maintain contact with the participants, be responsive to facial and body cues, and use the prompts, without providing solutions.

> Graduates of the program have demonstrated high satisfaction with the quality of the program, improved understanding of fall risk factors and prevention, and substantial follow-through of the behavioural steps designed to minimise the risk of falls.[19]

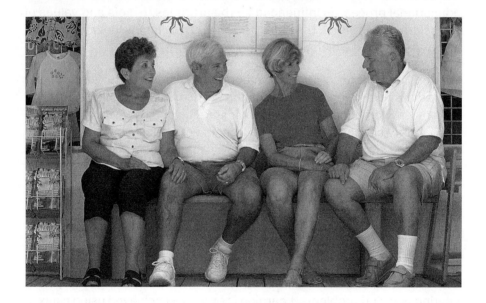

SELF-EFFICACY BELIEFS AS A TOOL FOR CHANGE

Self-efficacy is about people's expectations of their personal ability to function well in specific situations. The concept of self-efficacy is derived from Bandura's social cognitive theory.[20] What people are capable of achieving and what they actually do achieve is mediated by their sense of self-efficacy. Thus, a positive belief in one's personal ability is central to motivation and action.

---

19   Strommen, Brotherson, & Yang, 2017.
20   Bandura, 1977; Bandura, 1986; Bandura, 1997.

Increasing a person's self-efficacy has been shown to be a powerful tool in initiating and changing healthy behaviour.[21] For example, a belief about the need to exercise and about ability to engage in exercise can predict exercise participation.[22] A study by Cheal and Clemson[23] qualitatively evaluated the benefits of perceived self-efficacy in risk situations in a falls prevention program. That study highlighted the value of using techniques such as mastery experiences and verbal support to achieve activities such as safe bus travel.

Bandura[24] outlines four main types of influences on self-efficacy:

1. enactive mastery experiences (accomplishments)
2. vicarious experiences (the influences of others)
3. verbal persuasion
4. physiological and emotional states (messages from our bodies and feelings).

1. Enactive mastery experiences

Enactive mastery experiences are the most influential on behavioural change. Mastery is about doing, about success and failure, and about overcoming barriers. It is developed by practice, which can be assisted by breaking skills down into easily mastered subskills. The participants need to be clear as to how to carry out the safety behaviours correctly, and to understand the rationale behind their actions. Telling others about personal progress enhances self-efficacy and gives valuable self-satisfaction.

Breaking skills down into easily mastered subskills can help in the learning of safety behaviours. For example, a daily activity like walking is separated into easily mastered subskills. A shuffle walk is first demonstrated as an example of a risky behaviour. Defensive walking such as a heel-and-toe walk is demonstrated by the facilitator and explained step by step.

Barriers to follow-through need to be recognised, and strategies for overcoming the barriers developed. Repetition is also important: the exercises are repeated in the same format each week, including repeated explanations as to why the exercises work, as well as practice of particular exercises by request.

---

21 Bandura, 1995; Strecher, McEvoy DeVellis, B., et al., 1986.
22 Strecher, McEvoy DeVellis, B., et al., 1986.
23 Cheal & Clemson, 2001.
24 Bandura, 1986.

As strength and balance improve, safe walking skills can be more easily mastered, and the link between the skills and the gaining of strength and balance is taught. Additional discrete walking skills are added throughout the program, with people learning how to scan ahead to be aware of hazards like changes in level or uneven pathways, and to adjust their step or avoid them. A barrier to learning this skill could be an individual assuming 'scanning ahead' has to be done at all times, not realising that looking down is important upon reaching the hazard. For others, a lack of opportunity for walks and practice presents a barrier to the acquiring of new safety skills.

The program gives homework which is an essential part of the process of change and must be followed up in the following session. The facilitator needs to strive to become aware of personal accomplishments, and providing positive feedback week to week.

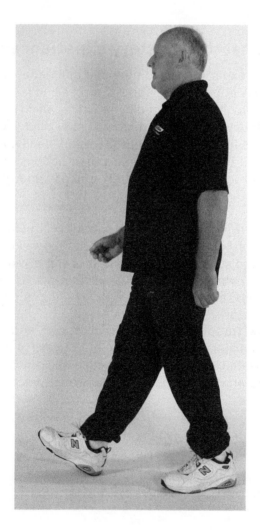

Jean was 94. She had retired in her early 80s from a successful private practice. She was interested to learn that it was possible to improve balance and worked very hard at this. She showed improvements within the first few group meetings, and other group members noticed the changes. Jean was visibly proud of her achievements. She would never accept that growing old meant that she had to accept physical problems. During the final meeting, when the group was reflecting on the program, many of the group members commented on how Jean had inspired them and helped them to try different approaches. Jean noted how she had gained in many ways and found the many everyday safety suggestions helpful (such as looking for a lamppost or something similar to hold on to for support as she stepped down the kerb when crossing the street). She said it was the demonstrations and clear explanations that had helped her to absorb new information so that she understood what to do and how to do it. Jean practised, followed through, and shared her accomplishments.

2. Vicarious experiences

Vicarious experiences can alter efficacy beliefs. The experience of observing others, who provide their own examples of competencies and attainments, can impact on how personal capabilities are appraised. The group process exposes participants to potential role models as stories are shared about safety-enhancing or risk-taking experiences. A role model is someone seen to be in similar circumstances, or even having similar personal characteristics. Role models can teach different ways of doing things, thus strengthening personal beliefs. They may emerge from the participants, their families and peers, or from the group facilitators and presenters.

3. Verbal persuasion

Positive social persuasion to tackle achievable goals can encourage people to try harder, and the facilitator has a role in demonstrating positive verbal support and in encouraging group members to support one another. Gage et al.[25] note how therapist encouragement and genuine optimism is infectious. In the group setting, this attitude quickly spreads, and the group process then works to provide peer support.

---

25 Gage, Cook & Fryday-Field, 1997.

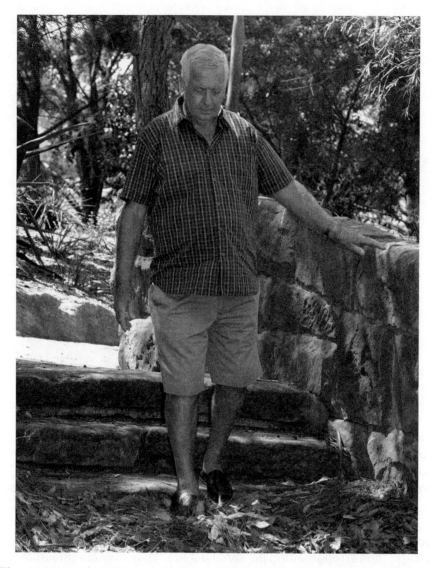

The opinions of significant others can result in sustained efforts. We have found that, for some people, including a spouse or friend in the program has been invaluable. Often people say they have shared ideas from the program with friends and people in other community groups to which they belong. This is very helpful to the people themselves, since sharing what is learned with others can be another source of reinforcement and part of the process of exploring options. In addition, teaching what is learned to someone else helps clarify what has been learned.

Erica emerged as a popular role model in one of our programs. She was a strong and intelligent lady who was caring for her husband (who had Alzheimer's) and a son (who had schizophrenia). She was active in community organisations, but found time to join the program to learn how she could reduce her risk of falling. She always asked useful questions and provided many insightful comments, which encouraged the group members to problem-solve. We all respected her as a role model. She actively put into practice the exercises and many of the other safety strategies that involved small but habitual changes. For example, coming down the stairs she noticed how her flowing pants caused her to trip. She shared how she was now grasping them out of the way as she went up and down her stairs and was rethinking the style of some of her clothes. At the follow-up group, she said she was still doing most of the exercises. When, while watching television with her granddaughter, she suddenly started raising her legs to do her nightly routine, her granddaughter began giggling. Erica was embarrassed and stopped the exercise. This was a case of negative verbal persuasion. The group responded with suggestions for humorous retorts to the granddaughter, and Erica began to regain her usual sense of control and to think about how she could handle the situation next time.

4. Physiological and emotional states

People use information from their physiological and emotional states to judge their capabilities. The impact of bodily responses can be quite powerful and should not be overlooked. We have had many people tell us that they felt they were making gains from the exercises, because they felt stronger or their balance was better. They were able to describe everyday activities that they found they could do more easily than before, like standing up or dressing. This was highly motivating for them. However, people need to be able to interpret bodily states correctly. They need to be able to tell when pain may be harmful and when an alternative exercise is necessary, or when soreness is temporary and only means that they are making gains.

Affective responses can influence how people judge their personal efficacy. Pleasant experiences can heighten beliefs about coping, whereas stress and agitated states are not conducive to developing self-efficacy and a sense of personal accomplishment. Moderate arousal of emotions can, however, be useful.

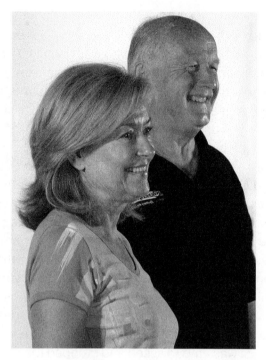

In summary, understanding how to work with the concept of self-efficacy and the factors that influence changes in efficacy beliefs will help to provide opportunities for change. This can result from the way material is taught, or by helping people to reflect on and reframe their experiences in positive but realistic ways. Most importantly, enhanced self-confidence in specific risk situations can lead to action and skill that can result in safer performance and better outcomes.

Remember

The facilitator has a responsibility to develop empathy, trust and a non-judgemental professional relationship with and among the participants. This will support the older person in adjusting their efficacy beliefs and help them to set their own realistic goals.

REFLECTIVE MOTIVATION, PROBLEM-SOLVING, AND FOLLOW-THROUGH OF SAFETY BEHAVIOURS

Early work reviewing medical and occupational safety research on compliance behaviour[26] found that the sustaining of falls prevention strategies depends on:

- the level of support (social and peer support)
- the ease of complying (cost/effort/complexity/intrusiveness)
- the technical competence and interpersonal skill of professionals
- the opportunity and willingness to undertake personal goal setting
- feedback about success.

Core to Stepping On is problem-solving, that is, assisting the participants to analyse their risks through prompts and a decision framework (the 'preventive framework'). This is followed by helping participants to explore strategies for overcoming barriers, and planning and reinforcement of behavioural and environmental changes.

This is a reflective process (called 'reflective motivation' by Michie, Atkins & West[27]), whereby intentions and planning are considered essential precursors to carrying out planned behaviours and making changes to routines. Reflective motivation leads to an understanding of why a particular safety strategy or exercise links to preventing falls, to improving safety and confidence, and to continued independence. There are many opportunities that arise throughout each session of Stepping On for the participants and the facilitator to make such links, building a desire for change. The program uses a range of techniques to facilitate active follow-through and sustained changes. As recognised in the systematic review by Kwasnicka et al.,[28] it is important that the behaviour is relevant to the participants and that it fits with their sense of identity. Practical and effective strategies for overcoming barriers to embedding the strategies in everyday life are learned, and there is a supportive group environment.

The program uses techniques such as:

- breaking goals into simple steps

---

26 Cole, Berger, & Garrity, 1988.
27 Michie, Atkins, & West, 2014.
28 Kwasnicka, Dombrowski, et al. 2016.

- encouraging participants to engage in the problem-solving process taking place in the group
- using cues that will remind participants to do the exercises (e.g. waiting for the kettle to boil can prompt them to remember to do their balance exercise; leaving the weights and manual by their favourite chair can remind them to do other exercises)
- defining target behaviours in concise and relevant ways (e.g. 'removing clutter from pathways' is the solution, but the actual behaviour required is being aware of potential clutter, such as shoes, and then working out where to put the clutter out of the way)
- reinforcing through peer group support, self-feedback and making it fun.

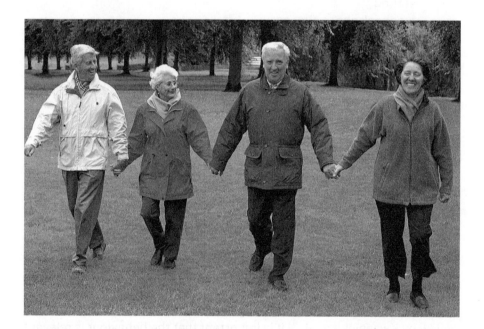

People use different cues as prompts for remembering safety strategies; for example, the start of a radio or TV program to do their exercises. This is consistent with habit theory, in which everyday events or situations can act as automatic prompts to action.[29] Thus, the intent, the planning, and repetition of the activity in the same context are all parts of changing a habit.

The facilitator needs to allow enough time to share, process and reflect on stories. Habits take time to change, which is why the sessions go over

29 Lally & Gardner, 2013, Clemson & Munro, 2016.

seven weeks, and why there is a three-month follow-up session. Homework needs to be followed up by the facilitator each week as part of a positive and optimistic review of what has been achieved, what has worked and how obstacles have been overcome. Checking the participants' checklists and weekly exercise records is also essential for reinforcement of individual progress in risk management.

This program is effective in assisting older people to gain a greater awareness of falls risk factors, explore different coping behaviours, and follow through on safety strategies in everyday life. We know that, if conducted correctly, Stepping On reduces falls in older people.

Stepping On group work, and the facilitator as a catalyst for change

Group work involves creating group cohesiveness as well as a good learning environment. People come together to share knowledge for personal development or to learn from one another through discussion. As Jacques and Salmon[1] describe, a group learning environment is one that allows the group members to draw on 'knowledge from outside the group in order to process it within, and subsequently use it outside.' The facilitator has a responsibility to select appropriate knowledge and supervise the processing of that knowledge in the group setting. It is important to ensure that participants draw upon their own backgrounds and experiences, so that the effects of the work done within the group endure beyond the program.

Even though we are highly connected through digital media, we can be disconnected from authentic experiences. Group work is about social interaction and engagement. The facilitator models expected behaviours, is forthright but non-judgemental, and has a genuine interest in the participants. The facilitator must understand that falls are preventable in older people. Facilitators need to assist discussion by using questioning, listening, and responding techniques.[2] They need to prompt, asking questions that help clarify, and explain key points. Good listening skills involve hearing what the person is saying and understanding the point that is being made, at the same time noticing what is transpiring in the group (all of which takes a great deal of energy). Responding can take the form of silence, prompts (questions), reflective statements, or praise. Above all, the facilitator encourages participants' questions and responses. Rather than telling the older person what they should do, it is more helpful to encourage them to reframe their story by asking questions, while actively listening.

The group belongs to the participants, who need to feel a sense of ownership of it. The facilitator validates the participants and helps them to

1   Jacques & Salmon, 2008.
2   Brookfield & Preskill, 1999.

develop a sense of trust. Chalk[3] outlines the following points about group work, all of which can be applied to the Stepping On program:

- A cohesive group focuses on a shared interest or concern. The first time the group meets is a very important opportunity for the participants to share their reasons for having joined the program.
- Information being provided is carefully balanced with opportunities for self-help, such as finding solutions to problems that have arisen in the participants' own day-to-day lives. The facilitator listens to the questions participants ask and to solutions they contribute, asks questions and then build on what the participants know. This is far more effective than simply giving out information.
- Facilitators will be most productive if they work with the group process. Health professionals are accustomed to giving expert advice; it is tempting to offer valuable information, and it is easy then to slip into a didactic lecturing style rather than being facilitative. However, it is important to recognise the expertise of all participants, to draw from their experiences, and to allow them to share and develop knowledge. For example, 'Mrs Smith made some wonderful points. Does anyone have anything to add?' It is much more empowering for group members to have the opportunity to come up with the ideas and find solutions, rather than simply to receive information. The role of the facilitator is to build the participants' sense of self-worth and their confidence in their own ideas and abilities.
- Learning to observe and maximise the group process is an acquired skill that comes with practice. Developing listening skills is a lifelong learning process. Debriefing with a co-facilitator can help to hone observation and group skills.
- The facilitator has an important responsibility to be aware of problems that might disrupt the flow of communication, interaction, and purposeful activity.
- Communication is central to group process and effective outcomes. This includes checking that intended meanings are understood by everyone, and that technical language and jargon is minimised. Avoid using jargon. Language needs to be simple and clear.

All of us have personal space and comfort zones in relation to others. Introduce people as they come to the group, always arrange seating

---

3   Chalk, 2000.

in a horseshoe where people can see one another, with chairs equally spaced, and establish that sessions will start and finish on time. Mobile phones need to be turned off, and laptops and other computers are not to be brought to the group. The facilitator stays with the group during all segments including guest segments.

It is vital to provide adequate opportunity for participants to contribute. Remember, the participants are thinking 'What's in this for me?' Stepping On can offset some of the psycho-social aspects of ageing, because there are chances to re-engage and meet new people. If group members have helpers, ask them to participate in the group, and to share their experiences as well.

The facilitator's role

The facilitator's role is central to the functioning of the program. Facilitators need to be good listeners, well organised, and positive and knowledgeable about falls prevention, and to have skills in running a group. Ongoing commitment from the group facilitator is very important and is noticed by group members. The facilitator creates a special bond with each person and inspires hope and a positive attitude to ageing.

PREFERRED SEATING AND GROUP SIZE

The horseshoe is the preferred seating arrangement. This seems the most comfortable for both the participants and the facilitator, and it maximises communication across the group.

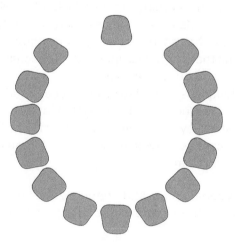

A circle works, but the horseshoe allows all participants to see and hear the facilitator equally well. It also gives space to display prompts, posters, etc.

The ideal group size is 12, so we often recruit 14 people, which allows for any absences. We always seem to have a few extras, as a close friend or spouse can join the program, and we include students, guest experts, and other visitors who come as 'participant observers'.

QUALITY FACILITATING

People have a natural desire to be social and connected and to have a sense of trust and belonging. Groups go through a number of stages between their beginning and ending. One model talks about storming, norming, performing and ending. For further reading refer to Jacques and Salmon.[4] Many of our participants have been socially isolated because of a fall or a fear of falling. Connection, laughter and fun can all be part of the group learning experience. Like all people, older people need social engagement.

Guest speakers are very important to the success of Stepping On. They provide the latest expert information and give the group the feeling that you value the participants enough to provide them with up-to-date advice.

The following tables summarise the activities associated with quality facilitating[5] and indicate what the facilitators of the group need to do for maximum educational effectiveness.

4   Jacques & Salmon, 2008.
5   Drawn from Bales, 1950.

Tips for initiating tasks[6]

INITIATE ACTIVITY	Initiate decision making and generate solutions. Take responsibility for introducing new topics, and the guest experts, in ways that motivate and arouse interest.
SEEK INFORMATION	Request information and ideas from participants. Ask them to clarify their suggestions.
GIVE INFORMATION	Give and ensure consistent and accurate information, and provide generalisations. The falls prevention facts must be correct, and consistent across all guest experts. This builds both trust and knowledge. Draw examples and stories from personal experience to illustrate points and stimulate sharing. The participants will want to know about their facilitator.
GIVE AND HEAR OPINIONS	State and reflect opinions and beliefs, taking notice of the values implied, not merely the facts. This is part of good listening.

6   Bales, 1950; Hare, Borgatta, & Bales 1965.

ELABORATE AND REFLECT	Clarify. Give examples and additional explanations to communicate the meaning or key point. The important points will be lost if mentioned only once and in only one session. Each session, ask participants to recall three points they remember from the previous session.
COORDINATE	The program needs to flow smoothly, so coordination is an important responsibility for the facilitator. There are many connecting ideas throughout the program, and it is necessary to show the relationships between the various ideas and suggestions. Making connections to personal contexts and situations and linking themes between topics will accelerate learning.
SUMMARISE	Summarise suggestions or ideas after discussion. Restate important points from the group's perspective.

Tips for successful maintenance of the group[7]

BE ENCOURAGING	Be friendly, warm, and responsive to the participants. Praise them and their ideas, and agree with and accept their contributions. Talk with them and never down to them. Respect them and their experiences. Always keep eye contact.
BE A GATEKEEPER	Assist everyone to contribute. Keep the program on track.
SET STANDARDS	Set and maintain group standards. These standards can be diverse and may include things like: one person speaking at a time; following up on homework from the previous week; encouraging questions and ensuring that the person who asks gets a response. The group members will take direction in this from the facilitator. Behave professionally and they will respect you: turn up on time, wear appropriate clothes, turn your phone off, and be cheerful.
SUMMARISE	Summarise the group reactions to ideas, and to feelings, if appropriate.

---

7   Bales, 1950; Hare, Borgatta, & Bales, 1965.

EVALUATE	See the final segment on evaluation in this chapter. Evaluation improves facilitation skills in the group process, as well as documenting and disseminating findings.
MEDIATE	See 'Working with different participant styles'.
RELIEVE TENSION	Draining off stress through a joke or a change of context can relieve tension that may develop in a group. The use of humour needs to be in context, people need to be able to connect with it, and it needs to be inclusive – the laughing needs to be 'with' and not 'at'. See below.
USE HUMOUR	Humour is a useful tool for making connections and learning. If shared, it is good for group cohesiveness. A sense of humour frequently appeared in our participants. The program was a great source of fun. Remember, laughter is the shortest distance between two people. FUN is so important. We have a natural desire to be social – and having a laugh lightens the mood and connects people.

WORKING WITH DIFFERENT PARTICIPANT STYLES

Some group members may exhibit behaviours that do not help the group to achieve its goals.[8] The facilitator needs to be able to recognise the reasons behind these behaviours. They are usually a symptom of an unmet personal need. The behaviours need to be managed in order for the facilitator to devote themselves more effectively to building group cohesion. It is useful to be aware that we all have different styles of interacting. Here, we make a few observations of ways in which we have learned to work with participants to develop a healthy group process. All styles were not always evident in every group.

The natural leader

Natural leaders are supportive of the facilitator. They usually sit themselves opposite the group facilitator (which is actually a good position for a co-leader). They also protect the group and do things like asking others to keep quiet in a timely and appropriate way.

The talker

The facilitator has to learn ways to keep the talker on the topic, and to quieten the talker politely when necessary. The group will appreciate the facilitator's dealing with disruptive behaviour. Talkers just need some attention, so give it to them in break times and before the group meeting begins. Talk to them and listen to what they have to say. Helpers and co-leaders in the group can do this as well. We have often used this strategy successfully.

The rebel

Once converted, the rebel is a valuable group member. It is important to take extra care to develop the rebel's trust in the first few group meetings. Rebels will put the leader to the test. They really want to know: 'What's in it for me? Am I wasting my time or is this really a valuable group?' Listen to what they say. Show that you know what you are talking about. Acknowledge what they are trying to say. But be open and honest and don't be afraid to tackle bad or disruptive behaviour. Other group members appreciate it.

---

8   Jacques & Salmon, 2008.

The submissive type

Submissive group members like to conform. They prefer being given direction to taking any personal control. They are the most difficult to engage, and extra attention at break times is helpful. The group approach needs to be inclusive, encouraging comments from everyone at different times; it may not be easy for submissive people to speak up, but it can be very valuable for them when they do participate.

The silent type

This type of participant is usually the best listener – still waters run deep! Try to draw them out gently. They often benefit more from the group than they appear to – even more so than the talkative ones because they are good listeners. They will do even better if they can share. Look for opportunities: they may talk to you or a co-leader at break times and share achievements. You may then be able to prompt them to re-tell some of these stories to the group.

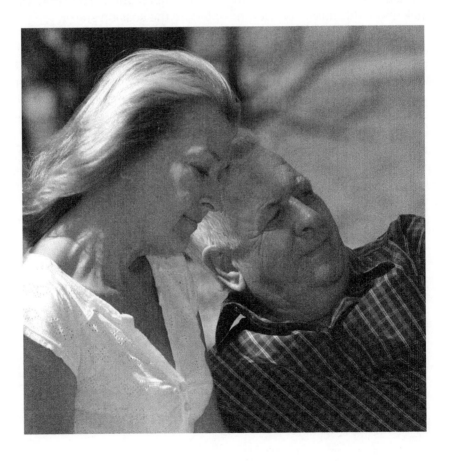

The joker

A joker can be a powerful aid to learning. Make sure the joking is inclusive of group members (i.e. is 'with' people and not 'at' anyone), and steer the jokes on to the topic. Listen to what the joker is saying and ensure you chat with them before the group.

The resistant type

The resistant person does not want to be there. We rarely encountered a person responding in this way in our programs. Attention to marketing and recruitment strategies (with clear explanations of the program) is important.

The preoccupied type

The preoccupied person is distracted for a reason. Is there a medical condition causing pain? Is eyesight or hearing making participation difficult? Is there a recent loss in their lives? Try to find out. An understanding of the reasons can help communication. They may want to talk about this during break time or before the session starts.

The complainer

Acknowledge the complainer's needs early in the program. We all need and want attention in different ways. The complainer commonly uses negative statements to gain attention, and this can contribute to their feeling down and believing that they lack control. Once again, use the strategy of listening to this person during break times. During group time, help such a person to reframe negative comments into positive statements. Though this can take time for the complainer, positive thinking can be learned and is conducive to health and wellbeing.

Key elements for delivery of Stepping On

The following is a list of key elements considered important or essential when delivering Stepping On. These elements were determined by a group of international experts using a modified Delphi technique.[1] The top five key elements were: (1) use plain language, (2) develop trust, (3) engage people in what is meaningful and contextual for them, (4) train participants in recognising cues to assist their self-monitoring of how they do the exercises, and (5) learn about the exercises and how to progress them.

ELEMENT	PERCENTAGE AGREEMENT
Adult learning: elements considered essential or very important	
Use plain language	100
Develop trust	100
Engage people in what is meaningful and contextual for them	100
Introduce yourself and ensure participants introduce themselves	94
Use optimism and positive talk	94
Link strategies and skills to personal goals	94
Facilitate engagement of all members of group	94
Ensure positive environment	90
Invite feedback	89

---

1   Mahoney, Clemson, et al., 2017.

Keep group focused	89
Use storytelling	89
Help break down solutions into simple steps	89
Use preventive framework	82
Slow pace	79
Use a variety of mediums to support learning styles	78
Invite group to suggest topics	72
Include discussion of last week's topics	72
Program: aspects considered essential or very important	
Final group evaluation in the last session	95
Objectives reviewed with group	89
Invited experts prepped ahead of time by facilitator	89
Facilitator reviews key messages from invited experts	89
The prior week's homework is reviewed each session	84
'Personal medication record card', with group discussion	84
Snacks and beverages	84
Group size of 10–14 participants	83
Homework is assigned each session	79
Topic handouts	74

Apple Game (i.e. knowledge quiz) with group discussion	74

Exercise: elements considered essential or very important

Train participants in cues for self-monitoring of how they do the exercises	100
Facilitator learns about the exercises and understands how to progress them	100
Facilitator links exercises to preventing falls	100
Facilitator shows where to buy or obtain weights, and how to put on ankle weights	95
Exercises are introduced in the first session	89
Facilitator has weights available at the class for participants to borrow	84
Each session includes some exercise	83
Introduce the concept of advancing exercises at the first session	77
Facilitator encourages 'snacking' on exercises	72
Facilitator collects exercise homework	72
All exercises in the manual are taught	62
Exercises are limited to those included in the manual	33

Upgrading exercise: elements considered essential or very important

Facilitator learns about the exercises and how to upgrade them	100
Facilitator believes that upgrading exercise is important	96

Facilitator encourages participants to advance exercises, as able, throughout the sessions	94
Facilitator teaches the participants the importance of challenging their balance (in Session 1)	89
Facilitator has strong self-efficacy that he/she can safely progress the exercises	89
Facilitator encourages participants to advance to not holding on during an exercise, as able, throughout the sessions	88
Facilitator encourages the use of weights, as able, throughout the sessions	78
Home visit: elements considered essential or very important	
Assistance with follow-through of falls prevention strategies and activities	100
Reinforcement of those falls prevention activities that have been accomplished	100
Support, and if necessary, assistance with putting into practice the safety strategies learned related to the home and community environment	95
Assistance with referral to support services (upon request)	89
Providing a session face-to-face in the home (as opposed to over the phone)	89
Assistance with home adaptations and modifications, if required	78
Supplementation of participant's assessments of falls hazards in and about the home	77
Booster session: elements considered essential or very important	
Objective of reviewing exercise barriers and strategies for overcoming barriers	95

Importance of the booster session itself	94
Objective of reviewing changes that have been put into practice	88
The timing of the booster session is at three months	59

Facilitator's role: elements considered essential or very important	
Facilitator develops a sense of ownership of the group by the participants	100
Facilitator inquires about and accommodates needs related to vision or hearing impairment	95
Facilitator debriefs with the co-leader after each class	95
Facilitator is skilled at interpreting themes and reframing ideas	89
Facilitator provides monitoring and feedback to invited expert regarding getting across key messages, using relevant examples, using group process, using plain language	89
Facilitator understands the concept of 'targeting the behaviour for change'	84
Facilitator provides instruction to the key expert before they meet with the group	84
Facilitator is skilled in prompting 'storytelling'	83
Facilitator is skilled in 'storytelling'	78
Facilitator is skilled in using the preventive framework	78
Facilitator calls people who miss a session	78
When leading, the facilitator presents himself or herself as equal with the participants in the group	56

Background and training of the facilitator: elements considered essential or very important

Facilitator has the ability to work with older people (i.e. experience and understanding of their needs)	100
Facilitator has a good knowledge of exercise	94
Facilitator has a good knowledge of falls prevention topics	94
Facilitator has previous experience with facilitating adult groups	88

Background of facilitator: other than a physical therapist, registered nurse, or occupational therapist, professions that could definitely or probably fulfil the role of facilitator

Retired physical therapist, occupational therapist	83
Social worker	82
Allied Health assistant	76
Health educator	76
Fitness expert	76
Non-professional peer leader	64

Co-leader's role: elements considered essential or very important	
Prompting questions	71
Role modelling how to be an active participant in the class	70

Background of invited expert who introduces exercises: professions that could definitely or probably fulfil the role	
Fitness expert	94
Allied Health assistant	89
Health professional with exercise training or exercise experience with older adults	88
Occupational therapist	76

Recognising culture

Culture is an important aspect of learning. It influences how we perceive or make sense of the world around us and how we respond or adapt to that ever-changing world. This world includes not only the physical environment, but also, perhaps especially, the people and social relationships within it. Culture, through communication and other behaviours, is significantly involved in developing trusting, rewarding relationships with people. Facilitators running groups in a language other than English need to find out about how the culture may affect beliefs and values in relation to falls, exercise, and the group environment. Adaptations may be needed.[1]

Culture, as a way of perceiving and responding to the world around us, can be an important factor both in falls and falls prevention, since what people see as a risk is influenced by culture. People in different age groups, for cultural and personal reasons, may see different circumstances as potential risks. As we age, we do not always recognise that our risk factors may change. This is often related to people's concept of self, another aspect that is influenced by culture. People's perceptions of risk and of barriers to changing behaviour can be influenced by both culture and personal experience.

Communication is inherently cultural. The language and communication styles we employ are influenced by culture – and these can vary quite significantly across cultural groups and age groups. The way we communicate with peers is often quite different from the way we communicate with others, particularly in formal (the session) or semi-formal (coffee break) situations. Cultural issues, like respectful behaviour and what is appropriate in certain contexts, often come into play. Introduction activities may need to be adapted for some groups in which using personal names or talking about oneself is considered inappropriate, or even rude or embarrassing. Asking direct questions may be offensive to people from some cultural groups. It may be necessary to consult with people from the target group to find ways to accomplish the aims in a more culturally appropriate and acceptable manner. All cultural groups have their own ways of getting to know others, and it could be valuable to draw upon some of these techniques, especially in multicultural groups, to add variety and interest.

1   Jang, Clemson, et al., 2015.

Storytelling or narration can be a very important cultural and communication event, since it is one of the most common ways in which people communicate. Not only is storytelling generally an enjoyable way to communicate, it presents an effective method of conveying difficult ideas, concepts, and emotions.

Finally, many of the theories we have about people – how they behave, what they need to learn, and how they will respond – are influenced by culture. Most of the ideas, theories, and experiences that provide the foundation for this program come from work with people from particular cultural backgrounds – that is, mainly white, middle-class Americans and Australians, primarily from or influenced by a Western cultural background. Thus, while the theories and ideas are important and have proved useful for these populations and others that are similar in many ways, it cannot be assumed that they are valid for all people from all cultural backgrounds. For example, ideas about self-efficacy are apparently valid for many cultural groups, but just what self-efficacy means, how it is played out, and how it is valued, can vary across cultural groups. Concepts like mastery may mean very different things in different populations.

Facilitators need to be culturally competent in their presentation of the program. In fact, the success of the program in any context is dependent on its cultural relevancy and sensitivity.

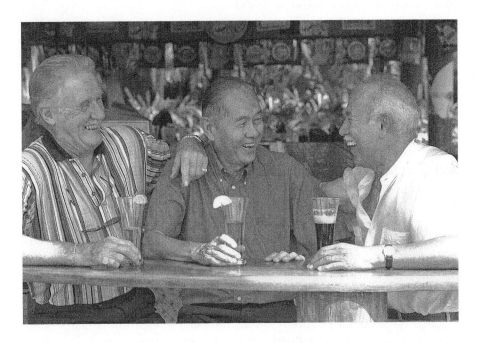

FACILITATING STEPPING ON FOR PEOPLE FROM CULTURALLY AND LINGUISTICALLY DIVERSE (CALD) BACKGROUNDS

Interviews with Stepping On program providers illustrate how there are extra layers of complexity involved in program planning, delivery, recruitment, and enabling participation of older people from CALD backgrounds.[2] There is a strong tradition that CALD program facilitators extend themselves, 'going the extra mile' to ensure a successful program. This includes consideration of how to reach and deliver the program to older people from CALD backgrounds, understanding the nuances of facilitation and participation, and locating additional resources.

Having a bilingual Stepping On facilitator can create an atmosphere that encourages learning using culturally appropriate approaches. Such facilitators can understand the experiences of the participants, enabling the older people to bring their own perspectives and knowledge to the group. They eliminate the need for interpreters, and this makes interaction and decision making easier. They can increase the likelihood of having culturally appropriate venues, catering and guest speakers, and build partnerships with local cultural organisations (which can assist with recruitment and the referral process).

Potential cultural adaptations

It is important to understand the participants' cultural backgrounds and their attitudes to ageing. For example, do they expect to be looked after by their children or grandchildren? Are they intending to retire? What are their attitudes and beliefs towards exercise?

Be aware of different cultural approaches to teaching and learning, and how they may differ from the teaching principles underpinning the Stepping On program. For example, regarding 'falls prevention', do they prefer to be advised about what to do by experts? What are their expectations? Are they culturally familiar with storytelling or the written word, or is a more directive style of education expected and preferred? Having a bilingual facilitator and bilingual presenters would enable inclusivity and encourage discussion.

It needs to be considered whether there should be any variation in emphasis regarding the specific content of this manual. For example, the uptake of vitamin D is an issue for cultures whose dress covers their arms and head.

---

2   Jang, Clemson, et al., 2017.

The message of falls prevention may not be as prevalent in communities where a language other than English is the first language. People's length of time of settlement in Australia may influence their access to such programs, and newer communities may have more work to do to develop networks.

When interviewed by Jang et al.,[3] program facilitators identified that, with effort, they were able to gain knowledge and experience about CALD communities and their needs and concerns, and to adapt the program to individual community circumstances. Bilingual facilitators need to be trained in the conceptual framework behind Stepping On. It is our experience that those CALD facilitators who first observe a group conducted in English and have the opportunity to co-facilitate an English-speaking group before they conduct one in their own language are better able to understand what can and what should not be adapted.

Free translated handouts in various languages are available for download from Sydney University Press (sydneyuniversitypress.com.au/stepping -on-2019).

CALD populations may pose challenges with respect to screening and recruitment – see sydneyuniversitypress.com.au/stepping-on-2019 – CALD training.

In summary, we recommend:

- that the CALD facilitator is a bilingual speaker who is conversant with the cultural, health and educational background of participants
- that the facilitator attend formal Stepping On training, and co-facilitate a program in English before they start their own CALD Stepping On group
- that the guest speakers (physiotherapist, occupational therapist, vision expert, pharmacist, etc.) are bilingual
- that the CALD programs are planned and carried out in partnership with the local community
- that the program is properly planned and considered, so that it delivers value for money and achieves all the objectives.

---

3   Jang, Clemson, et al., 2017.

Marketing and recruitment

It is important to develop a marketing plan in the early stages. This will involve defining the size, geographical area, and other attributes of the primary target market, the most efficient methods of recruitment, and ways of sustaining the program over time. Outlined below are some methods that have been successful. (Note, your plan should include costs in terms of both time and money needed for marketing and recruitment.)

Outline the marketing and recruitment plan and identify:

- the primary target market
- resources for marketing materials
- the best methods of recruitment for the community
- resources for handling enquiries
- a financial budget
- ways of sustaining recruitment.

It appears that using just one recruitment method is not sufficient, and a variety of methods are required.[1] The kinds of recruitment strategies that have been most successful are media editorials and mail-outs using a computerised list. Recruit the assistance of a club, a general medical practice, an organisation, or perhaps a local council to undertake mail-outs. Media editorials can be cost-effective to initiate in a new area – we wrote our own editorials and sent them, with a photograph, to local newspapers. However, this cannot be sustained on a regular basis. Then other avenues are needed. One successful way of gaining new recruits is to send a letter to each participant's local doctor after graduation. This letter could outline that their patient successfully completed the program and what the program involved. See a suggested letter in the appendices.

Flyers or brochures distributed to community organisations can supplement the main recruitment strategy. A copy of one of our flyers is included as a suggestion. We sometimes found it extremely helpful to liaise with local council aged care workers as gate keepers to local organisations and activities. To be most cost-effective, make presentations to large gatherings and allow time afterwards to talk to individuals. A Health Fair held during 'Older People Week' worked well for us in one locality, but not in another.

---

1   Clemson, Taylor, et al., 2007; Garrett, Thomas, et al., 2000.

Volunteers for the groups can be asked whether their spouse or a friend wish to join the program. Having peers and spouses involved can assist with learning and support for the participant, and they may benefit themselves. Participants are sometimes an underused resource

---

Many older people have had a fall experience that has shaken their confidence and may have resulted in injury. Older people understand that the threat of a fall can be a barrier to safely doing all the things they want to do at home and to Stepping On confidently in the community. The prevention of falls is vital to maintaining personal independence.

WHY SHOULD I BE CONCERNED ABOUT FALLING

1. More than one third of adults 65 or over fall each year

2. Among older adults falls are the leading cause of injury, hospital admissions for trauma and death.

3. 35% of people who fall do less. Falls can reduce mobility and independence

FALLS PREVENTION

Stepping On is a well researched falls prevention program. The results were published in the September 2004 issue of the American Geriatrics Society.

Stepping On

Building Confidence and Reducing Falls

An effective program for older people

Logo of partner organization
Address/ contact details

Stepping **On**

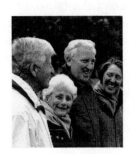

Stepping On

WHAT IS COVERED

- Balance and strength training
- Vision and falls
- Medication and falls
- Pedestrian safety and falls
- Safe footwear
- Home safety

WHAT WILL I DO

Attend the program for two hours a week for seven weeks followed by a refresher session three months later.

The program is part of a research project and we will ask you to complete a survey before and after the program and test your mobility.

'When I'm walking I still have to think, "lift your feet, walk heel–toe". I have stopped falling outside! It has made me more aware of the way I walk.'
Grace

'I've had some near falls but you have a quicker recovery and your muscles don't collapse.'
Herbert

WHO PRESENTS

The program is led by:_____

_____

Health professional experts also assist with the program. Local experts include a physiotherapist and occupational therapist from the local area health service, a vision expert and a medications expert.

WHERE

Programs will be starting:_____

Venue:_____

_____

Transport: If you have difficulty with transport, let us know.

WHO CAN JOIN

Any one who is:

- 65 years or over
- Had a fall in the past year
- Fearful of falling
- Living at home
- Not suffering from dementia

PHONE:

'Its made me more aware, just so much more aware. Of the buses, of my place. Of making it brighter inside, getting rid of leaves outside, of everything.'
Roleena

BENEFITS

- Learn to step outside your home with confidence
- Learn with your peer group
- Become more aware of fall hazards and that fall risk can be reduced
- Up-to-date information of falls prevention
- Take control back into your life

HOW TO REGISTER

I am interested in attending Stepping On. Please contact me:

Name:_____

Phone number:_____

Address:_____

_____

for marketing the program, but once the programs are underway, the participants may assist by recommending the program to others. Flyers could be available in sessions, for participants to take if they wish to assist with recruitment. Word of mouth is a very powerful marketing tool.

With their permission, a photo of a former participant, with some personal comments, is the best advertisement for the program. We included a copy of the article in some of our mail-outs, and a blow-up of it on a poster at presentations. These items have proved to be the best way of explaining what the program is about.

Additional media avenues could include paid advertising and local radio. We suggest that an advertisement might be more successful if, like the editorial, it includes a photo and some remarks from a former participant.

One of the factors that influences recruitment is the venue, the most desirable venue being one in a central location accessible by public transport. If the location has difficult access (e.g. if the surrounding streets are steep), or if it is more than about 15 kilometres away from a local centre, it may be less popular. The day of the week on which the sessions are held is important to many people, and being able to offer the program on various days is an advantage. Avoiding holidays is desirable. Morning groups work well.

Have information regarding community transport in the area.

Remember, WORD OF MOUTH is the most powerful form of marketing and recruitment. Ask your Stepping On participants to talk about the Stepping On program to their GPs/health providers. Send letters to GPs/health providers regarding their patients' participation in the program.

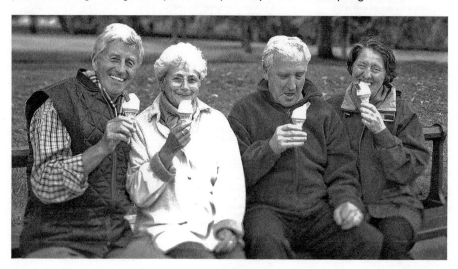

Evaluation

Evaluation can provide important information to ensure that the program is conducted as intended and that the core elements are maintained. Key factors to evaluate are:

1. the nature of the intervention (process), including coaching tools (sometimes referred to as 'fidelity checks')
2. the effects on the participants (impacts)
3. the longer-term consequences (outcomes).

THE NATURE OF THE INTERVENTION (PROCESS)

Evaluating the intervention and its process is an appropriate starting point in establishing the quality of the program; such evaluation asks whether the group process is happening effectively, and whether the activities and approaches are covering the content adequately. As programs are rolled out, adaptations are needed for local contexts, and program 'drift' can occur in which core elements needed for success are changed or eliminated. This is why the use of fidelity tools can be so important.

The core elements for Stepping On were established through a Delphi consensus process with experts from the United States of America, Canada and Australia.[1] For example, the experts supported the prime components of the conceptual underpinning of the program (adult learning theory and behaviour change) as essential. The principles of self-efficacy were rated as highly important, and decision making (the preventive framework) was rated as important. They affirmed the need for facilitators to have skills in these concepts and in group work, and to have evidence-based knowledge of falls prevention. They also acknowledged the importance of understanding and applying other key program elements (as previously discussed), especially the upgrading of exercises.

From the Delphi process and subsequent focus groups with stakeholders, Stepping On fidelity (or coaching) surveys have been developed to provide reflective tools for facilitators and trainers. The tools have been used to generate a checklist of core elements indicating that the program is being

---

1   Mahoney, Clemson, et al., 2017.

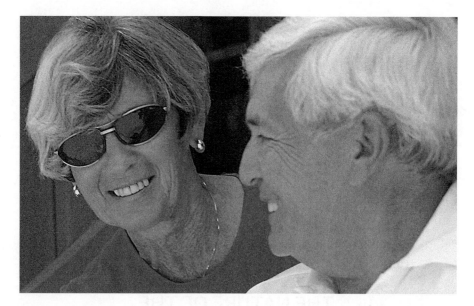

run as intended. The evaluation involves reflecting on how the program is being delivered by the facilitator, and on how it is being received and applied by the participants.[2] The tools can be used through self-reflection (by the facilitator and the participants) or through observation (by peers or experts).

The coaching/fidelity tools can be used when training facilitators and when delivering Stepping On. During training and delivery, the aim is to identify lapses in fidelity and to validate the strengths and the quality of the program. Like a builder's hammer, an evaluation tool has to be used correctly. It requires adequate feedback and thoughtful reflection, not just the mechanical filling out of a form. It seeks to establish which core elements are being incorporated effectively and should be continued, and how other elements could be applied in a different way or strengthened. Below are examples of the tools, reproduced with permission of the Wisconsin Institute for Healthy Aging.

The fidelity tools are available from www.steppingon.com

Other evaluations that can measure enactment include simple attendance data, or a survey of participants to investigate the extent to which the program has helped the respondents from their own perspective.

---

2   Carroll, Patterson, et al., 2007; Robb, Burns, et al., 2011.

Sample of items from the Session 3 Fidelity Coaching Tool.

EVENT	RATE QUALITY	COMMENTS
	0 = Not done at all 1 = Not satisfactory 2 = Satisfactory 3 = Very satisfactory 4 = Excellent	
Balance and strength exercises were practised, with the facilitator concentrating on exercises with which people had trouble.	0 1 2 3 4	
All exercises were linked to the reasons for doing them and how the exercises prevent falls.	0 1 2 3 4	
Facilitated the discussion about home falls hazards using Microsoft® PowerPoint or handouts of slides.	0 1 2 3 4	
PROCESS		
Facilitator invited feedback throughout.	0 1 2 3 4	
Facilitator demonstrated skill in using reflective listening.	0 1 2 3 4	
Participants told falls or safety strategy stories.	0 1 2 3 4	

Questions can include:

1. What was most useful?
2. What was least useful?
3. What is one thing you have used from last week?
4. What could be done differently?
5. What do you think about the venue and the timing?

The facilitator can evaluate and enhance their own skills in the group process: after a session it is instructive to write down what went on, how participants communicated and responded, how they contributed, how the guest speaker was received, what the participants seemed to be learning, and how this was demonstrated. It is also useful to ask someone else to observe the same group and take notes, and to compare and discuss the findings. How could things be done better? What really worked? Who has individual needs that require attention? This process will help improve observational and group work skills.

THE EFFECTS (IMPACTS) ON THE PARTICIPANTS

The questions here relate to the initial effects of the program in achieving its aims and session objectives. Has it made an impact? Have participants made any changes to their exercise habits? Have they implemented safety strategies at home and in the community? Are they using the 'Personal medication record card' to help with medication reviews? Have they had their eyes tested? Do they feel more confident doing things they previously were concerned about for fear of falling? Do they access the community more? Have they improved their social networks and contacts (if this is a goal for your participants)? Do they feel more in control?

Some examples include:

1. The timed 'Get Up & Go Test' is a validated measure of gait and mobility. It can easily be administered in any setting and is a useful measure for demonstrating gains both to the participants themselves and to the facilitator. The test records the time taken to get up from a chair, walk at a safe and comfortable pace for three metres (ten feet), turn around, walk back and sit down again.[3] It must be administered in exactly the same way before and afterwards so true comparisons can be made.
2. The 'Near Tandem Stand Test' measures how long the participant can stand in a near tandem stance, with eyes closed, testing for up to ten seconds. Older people tend to like this test because it

---

3   Mathias, Nayak, & Isaacs, 1986; Podsiadlo & Richardson, 1991.

can show how their balance has improved; however, when they start it reinforces how they need to improve their balance.

3. The 'Falls Behavioural Scale for Older People'[4] (FaB) was developed for Stepping On and can provide a baseline falls risk assessment before the program (or the particular behavioural changes), then be repeated after the program (or the behavioural changes). It can be downloaded freely from: www.fallspreventiononlineworkshops.com.au/resources

4. Other useful tests are the Falls Efficacy Scale – International (FES-I).[5] The FES-I is an assessment of a person's self-efficacy or confidence that they will not fall in specific circumstances. It is available in numerous languages. There are other self-efficacy scales, such as the Modified Falls Efficacy Scale (MFES),[6] which shows changes in confidence in mobility situations, and the Iconographical Falls Efficacy Scale (Icon-FES), which uses pictures to assess fear of falling in a range of activities and situations,[7] and is available as an app for mobile and tablet devices.

5. QuickScreen, developed by a team led by Tiedemann,[8] is a multifactorial clinical tool designed specifically for use as a screening tool for detecting falls risk; however, it also demonstrates considerable ability to detect change in physical status over time.

THE LONGER-TERM CONSEQUENCES (OUTCOMES)

Investigating the longer-term consequences answers the bigger-picture outcome questions that relate to the ultimate goals of the program. If facilitators and participants achieve the objectives – implement the safety strategies and do the exercises – will the participants then achieve the goals of reducing falls and improving their quality of life? These questions are best answered in rigorous randomised trials with long-term follow-ups and control comparisons.

We do not suggest evaluating the program by monitoring falls, but it may be useful to monitor individuals who continue to have recurrent and frequent falls. People who continue to fall frequently may require specific referral for medical, balance or neurological assessment (see Session 7 for more information on dizziness).

---

4   Clemson, Cumming, & Heard, 2003; Clemson, Bundy, et al., 2008.
5   Kempen, Todd, et al., 2007.
6   Hill, Schwartz, et al., 1996.
7   Delbaere, Smith, & Lord, 2011.
8   Tiedemann, Lord, & Sherrington, 2010.

Part 2

—

The Stepping On program

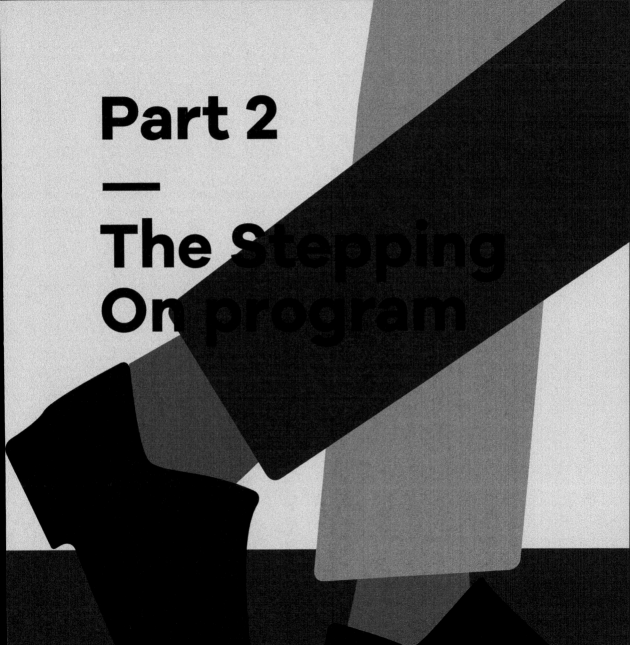

Stepping On overview

This section provides a quick overview of the program, information on preparing and planning for the program, and detailed outlines of the sessions, including the home visit and the three-month follow-up session. Each session outline begins with a list of the objectives that need to be achieved in that session. Time allocations are suggested for each segment, but flexibility will be needed within the overall constraints, because the time needed to adequately cover the material can vary from group to group. Homework is given to encourage active learning.

> A prerequisite to planning the program is to have read the 'Background' chapter. This chapter provides the group facilitator with the conceptual underpinning of the program and guides the way in which the program is to be delivered.

Sessions 1 and 2 are not flexible with respect to the guest speakers and topics to be covered. However, in the other sessions, the days on which topics can be presented are flexible. The timing can be arranged to suit the needs of the group. If a topic is not covered or not completed, it can be dealt with in the following session. Guest speakers are mandatory for the success of the program.

For information on each topic, it is essential to refer to the session chapters. Many sessions also have handouts and other resources, which can be found within the Sydney University Press website (sydneyuniversitypress. com.au/stepping-on-2019).

Quick overview of the program

SESSION 1   **Introduction, overview, and risk appraisal**

Build trust; provide an overview of program aims; encourage sharing of fall experiences; choose what to cover; and introduce the balance and strength exercises.

SESSION 2   **The exercises and moving about safely**

Review and practise the exercises; explore the barriers to and benefits of exercise; and discuss moving about safely with respect to chairs and steps, and learning not to panic after a fall.

SESSION 3   **Home fall hazards**

Identify fall hazards in and about the home; jointly find solutions to problems; and identify clothing hazards.

SESSION 4   **Community safety and footwear**

Generate strategies for getting around the local community with a reduced risk of falling; discuss the features of a safe shoe; and discuss strategies to assist with safe public transportation.

SESSION 5   **Vision, vitamin D, calcium and transportation safety**

Recognise the influence of vision on the risk of falling; review strategies to reduce the risk of falling from visual dysfunction; and identify the importance of vitamin D, sunlight and calcium to protect against fall injury.

SESSION 6	**Medication management and mobility mastery experiences**
	Identify the links between medications and the risk of falls; explore strategies for reducing the risk of falls from medication side effects or misuse; identify behavioural alternatives to taking sedatives for improving sleep; review exercises; review and further explore strategies for getting out and about in the local community safely; practise safe mobility techniques (learned during the program) in a nearby outdoor location.
SESSION 7	**Reviewing and planning ahead**
	Give participants the opportunity to talk about their personal accomplishments of the past seven weeks and to reflect on the scope of the things they have learned; review any areas requested; finish any segment not adequately covered; hand out graduation certificates; and allow time for farewells and closure.
	Home visit: Support follow-through of preventive strategies and assist with home modifications.
	Letter: Send letter to participants' local doctors
SESSION 8	**Three-month booster session:** Review achievements and discuss how to keep them going.
	Six-month booster session: Give a phone call at about six months to help sustain gains.

Preparing and planning for the program

SELECTING THE VENUE

Seeking out a suitable community-based venue is the first challenge. It needs to be accessible and close to public transport. Participants may need assistance with even small obstacles at the beginning of the course, but as they gain strength and confidence, they will want more independence. Ensure your venue is accessible and inviting, with enough room for all of the activities in each session. A large area is good, but too large will not create a good learning environment.

Checklist for venue selection

CHECK THE VENUE FOR SUITABILITY	
There is easy access to the meeting space.	☐
It is close to public transport.	☐
There is adequate signage marking the meeting space and the exits.	☐
There are accessible toilets, preferably with hand rails.	☐
There are enough chairs at the venue, preferably with arm rests.	☐
There is space for display tables and for practising exercises.	☐
There is access to electricity for the home hazard PowerPoint presentation if used and for boiling water for tea and coffee.	☐
There is no glare from the windows and it is not noisy. For example, avoid a venue next door to a children's play area, or where the type of floor makes hearing difficult.	☐

CHECK THE VENUE FOR SAFETY HAZARDS	
Make sure all exit signs are working properly.	☐
Make sure that fire alarms are working properly.	☐
Make sure there is a fire evacuation plan in order and that you are familiar with it.	☐
Check the floor for any trip hazards, including lifted carpet or electrical cables. You may need to tape these down to prevent tripping.	☐
CHECK THE TRANSPORT OPTIONS	
Ensure there is nearby public transportation, or that the venue has a private bus that can do pick-ups.	☐
You may need to arrange a hire bus. If this is needed, explore funding options within the local community.	☐
Is adequate parking available?	☐

Ensuring accessibility is paramount in the first few weeks, while the participants are still building confidence. Make sure the toilets are accessible and have handrails. It can be embarrassing for someone to have to ask for assistance in front of the other group members.

As you select the venue, make sure there are chairs and tables available, or that you can bring enough in from another location. When checking the furniture, consider: are the chairs suitable? Is there a choice of chairs? Can I get some with arms? Can I store chairs at the venue? Similar questions apply to any tables you might need. Make sure everything is safe and easy to use and move.

Ensure you have space to set up any displays. Having tables available at the venue is an advantage; otherwise, portable, foldable tables are a great alternative.

Name tags are a great way of making sure everyone knows who everyone else is. Also the guest speakers like to engage with participants and know their names. Having name tags in large print helps with reading, and collecting them at the end of each session will help make sure no one forgets to bring them.

Note: Follow up anyone who is absent – call to find out if there are any problems. People appreciate a call. At the beginning of the first session, ask people to let you know if they can't make any session. The group, as well as you, will like to know what is happening. The main reasons why people are absent are usually related to health, medical appointments or prearranged holidays. Participants then feel encouraged to take ownership of the group.

TRANSPORTATION

Some people need assistance to get to and from the class. This can vary from just one or two people to up to a third of the group. Plan for transport needs and use community services if available. You may want to develop a budget and explore funding options to provide transportation for those who need it, which may only be for the first few sessions while participants improve in mobility and gain confidence. Some venues, such as clubs, have their own transport buses.

THE ENVIRONMENT

The environment within the venue needs to be comfortable for the participants, but must also allow them to be engaged with the session and the facilitator. You will need to consider the special needs of your group. Get to know who has hearing or visual problems in Week 1, and do what you can to ensure they can get the full benefit from the program. Some people will need to sit closer to the facilitator and guest speaker.

Be aware of falls hazards in the venue – cords in walkways, and dimly lit rooms or bathrooms. Take some action to reduce or eliminate these hazards; you can be really obvious about it and use it as a learning experience with the group. Bringing duct tape for cords and extra lighting for dim areas can make all the difference.

Check that:

- the carpet is not torn or lifted
- all exits are marked
- any glass doors are clearly marked
- the floor is level and stable
- there is no debris in the walkways
- the venue is adequately lit
- there are no electrical cords in walkways
- the room is not too hot or too cold.

HEARING IMPAIRMENT

Identify the participants who have a hearing problem. Studies have shown that people will try to hide the fact that they have a hearing impairment. If you think someone does have a hearing impairment, but seems embarrassed about it, talk to them in private during the break and ask if they would like to be seated closer to where you are presenting.

Be alert and aware of external noises that might cause problems for people in the group. If you don't normally notice background noise, you will need to consciously think about it. To minimise the issue, you may need to shut the door and windows and situate the chairs away from a busy, noisy street.

Tips for talking to a person with a hearing impairment

- Make sure the person with the hearing impairment is seated where they can see your lips and the guest speaker's lips.
- Check that the light is shining on the speaker's face, not in the eyes of the person with the hearing impairment.
- Face the person with the hearing impairment directly and on the same level whenever possible.
- Establish eye contact.
- Speak in a normal fashion, without shouting or elaborately mouthing words.
- When you get the opportunity, find out whether they have (and are wearing) a hearing aid with batteries that work.
- Keep your hands away from your face while talking.
- Use gestures, body language and facial expressions to support what you say.
- Keep questions to a person with hearing impairment short and succinct.
- If you are eating or chewing while talking, your speech will be more difficult to understand.
- Recognise that people with a hearing impairment hear (and therefore understand) less when they are tired or ill.
- If a person has difficulty understanding some particular phrase or word, try to find a different way of saying the same thing, rather than repeating the original words over and over.
- Presenting visual prompts and providing written materials can supplement verbally delivered material.

VISUAL IMPAIRMENT

Loss of visual acuity is a common occurrence as we age, but some people become embarrassed about their diminishing sight. Keep an eye out for participants leaning forward and squinting, or asking the people around them to describe displays to them. If you think someone has visual impairment, talk to them in the break and ask whether they have any trouble seeing and if they have any glasses. It is also very likely that someone in your group will be sensitive to glare because of glaucoma, cataracts, or other visual problems such as macular degeneration. Moving the person to another seating position may help.

Tips for helping people who have a visual impairment

- Glare is a common problem, and you will need to take steps to reduce its impact.
  - Never seat people so that they have to look into the glare of a window or mirror.
  - If glare is a major problem in the environment, you may need to find some curtains or sheets to block some of the light.
- Use a large font for handouts, and contrasting, light-coloured paper with dark text.
- Do large writing in black felt pen on the flip charts. This gives more contrast.
- Give assistance when necessary at break time with snacks and beverages.
- Identify yourself and do not assume that participants will recognise you.
- Speak naturally and clearly. Loss of eyesight does not mean loss of hearing.
- In the group situation, cue a person with visual impairment into a conversation by mentioning their name.
- Tactile prompts are useful. Use relevant items from the display table.

SETTING UP THE VENUE

Items needed include chairs, tables, signage directing participants to meeting area, display items (according to session content), handouts, name tags and attendance sheets, break time foodstuffs, e.g. tea, coffee, sugar, biscuits, kettle, mugs/paper cups, and spoons.

Set up the room early. Be there for the early comers and to sort out transport or room problems. There is always at least one problem on the first day – that's Murphy's Law! Prepare signs directing participants to the room where the class will be held.

The most effective set-up is to have the chairs in a horseshoe with the facilitator or the guest facilitator at the head (see 'Preferred seating and group size' in 'Stepping On group work, and the facilitator as a catalyst for change'). This will enhance the group learning environment, because everyone will be in a good position to see and hear one another and the facilitator. If the room is too long and narrow, you are more likely to get two people talking at once. You also need room behind the chairs to practise the exercises.

Have the snacks and beverages set up for the break and the name tags ready near the doorway, along with an attendance list of names. The display of safety items will need a table as well, and there needs to be a spot on this table for the leg weights. Posters can be set up around the room.

BREAKS

Break times are just as important as the formal group time. The learning process is still going on; it is just more relaxed. This should be explained to your guests and visitors.

Some people may wish to talk with the facilitator because they have not heard or understood something, because they want to talk one-to-one about a personal issue, or because they wish to clarify or recap certain points. Break time is also an opportunity for participants to share stories about things that have happened to them and, especially as the group progresses, about what they are achieving. Having a co-facilitator, students, or other staff members present at break time may be helpful. Invite co-workers to join the group as much as possible. It can be an opportunity for them to learn about falls prevention and/or to develop confidence in group work. In addition, inclusion of the guest speaker in break time is a good way to get them more actively involved and to increase the participants' interest in what they have to say.

People tend to relax over a cup of tea or coffee and open up to one another, and this can mean it is a time when people will feel more comfortable about asking or answering questions.

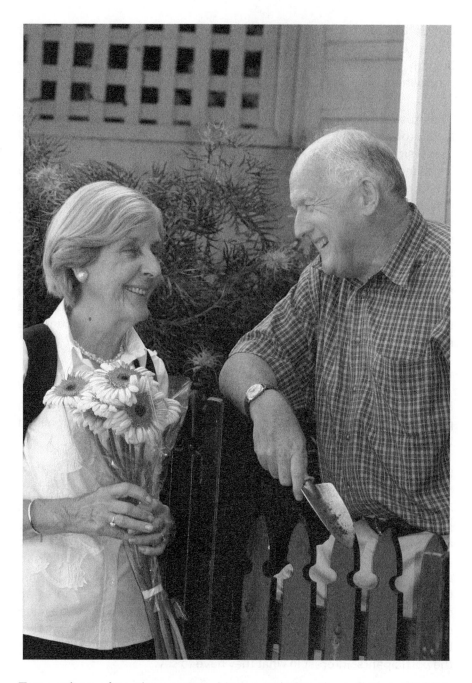

Two graduates from the program. Meg says, 'When I'm walking I still think, "Lift your feet, walk heel-and-toe!" I have stopped falling outside! It has made me more aware of the way I walk.'

John reported, 'I am much more aware of taking care and to walk properly with my walking stick. I feel stronger and more alive.'

Delivery of sessions

THE STEPPING ON FACILITATOR'S ROLE

The facilitator's role is central to the functioning of the program. Facilitators need to be good listeners, well organised, positive in attitude, and knowledgeable about falls prevention. Ongoing commitment from the group facilitator is very important and is noticed by group members. The facilitator creates a special bond with each person and inspires hope and a positive attitude to ageing.

The facilitator needs to maintain an up-to-date list of secondary contacts and ongoing referrals, and a supply of resources and brochures for additional services.

The facilitator may at times need to refer people on who are unsuitable for the program, e.g. to Parkinson's programs, dementia specific programs, outpatient physiotherapy classes and occupational therapy home visits.

> It is of great importance that the same facilitator remain with the group from beginning to end – changing facilitators during the seven weeks disrupts the development of trust and the flow of the program. Also, when guest speakers are present, the facilitator needs to remain part of the group – they need to reinforce the key messages. They also need to know that the guest speaker is on-topic. Behaviours by the facilitator such as leaving the room or checking a mobile phone are distracting and disrespectful.

The 'Background' chapter explains the responsibilities of the facilitator role and provides the information necessary for them to understand why the program runs the way it does, and to be able to answer questions as they arise. It also explains the significance of improving people's confidence about coping with fall risk situations, and provides information on how to improve self-efficacy. It describes the features of a good adult learning environment, and stresses the importance of respecting and building on the knowledge and skills of the participants. It outlines the decision-making process that will lead to falls prevention actions.

BEFORE THE SESSION
Preparing the guest speakers

These are people you have chosen because they have particular expertise. Prepare the guest expert with information on falls related to their topic. Each guest facilitator receives a copy of:

1. the session outline
2. the information in the program chapter pertaining to the delivery of their segment. This provides the key points and how the segment is conducted.
3. a copy of the Topics section from the session chapter that provides background to falls and their content area. This assists them to focus on the segment and be prepared for questions.
4. a copy of each of the supporting research articles
5. a copy of the Stepping On handouts.

Always meet with the guest facilitator prior to the program to explain the program philosophy and the format of the session.

Remind the guest facilitator to bring props or large photos as learning tools, e.g. spectacle cleaners; a large chart showing safe shoes; home safety devices such as touch lamps, etc. Do not use slide presentations as these disengage people; other than in the 'Home Falls Hazards' section, we have found that props and large picture charts work best.

Always provide feedback to the guest speaker following their session and thank them. Let them know if they did a great job of getting across key messages, and be up front if they drifted off-topic and did not stay relevant to falls prevention. Always provide particularly good feedback to each *new* guest expert, focusing on what worked and what they could do differently next time. They usually appreciate this. For example:

> 'Cover issues to do with pedestrian safety, as [you did] last time – crossing roads, safe clothing and being seen. We could leave out the bit on driving; I know you usually talk to others about this, but it is not the focus of this group, and we need to stay focused on falls issues. The bit on bag-snatching was good, but (if you don't mind) we do cover that in later sessions, so you can leave that out. That will give more time for … That was great!'

'The groups are very interactive, and we encourage discussion and lots of questions. It was great that you started to chat with people about your topic when they arrived and again at break. We find it is at these times that people digest and reflect on the safety strategies and validate, with you and each other, the important messages.'

If you have marketed the group well and the participants appreciate being part of the group and are actively learning, you will find that the guest speaker will enjoy the experience and be happy to return. Make sure that the group size is not too big or too small. Ask the guest speaker to stay for breaks, or if presenting halfway through, to come early so that they can join in the break and be available for answering questions. Mention that you give homework to be followed up the next week on key points from the session.

Sometimes requests for appointments to their services are made during break time.

The facilitator may prepare some open-ended questions related to the speaker's topic to stimulate discussion among participants at the start of the session.

The display

Learning can be better when using a variety of senses and experiences: hearing, looking, doing, feeling and touching. To enhance the learning in the program, use posters and a display of safety devices each week. The participants can browse before the group session and at break time (see 'Part 3: Resources' for suggestions).

The handouts

Participant handouts have been developed to provide key points for the different Stepping On topics and segments. These are not included in the manual but are available to be downloaded and copied for each participant. They are considered essential to the program. They should not be changed as they have been carefully prepared and based on evidence. They are copyrighted but can be freely reproduced with acknowledgement.

These include:

- A quick overview of the Stepping On program
- A one-page summary of each session
- 'Balance and strength exercise manual'
- The 'Shopping list' for Session 1.

There are also handouts of key points for most of the topics segments (e.g. 'Walking stick safety'; 'Products for slippery surfaces'; 'What is a safe, comfortable shoe'; 'Vision and falling' – and lots more).

We have found that some people use the handouts extensively and share them with friends or other groups to which they belong. This is very encouraging and helps in learning and follow-through of strategies. However, there is a danger of over-reliance on handouts on the part of the facilitator, because not everyone uses them. They are not to be relied on as the sole source of learning or reinforcement. It is good practice to hand out these information sheets at the end of the session, only to those interested, and one week at a time. Remember that some people cannot read well and others may have vision problems.

The handouts have been prepared as a review of the key messages for each topic. Reprint them on different coloured paper, but choose colours that are not too dark. A handy guide is that if you are unable to photocopy something successfully, it is too dark for some people to read.

Checking the safety of the environment

Every time you are about to begin a session, you should have a look around for any safety hazards. Do the check after you have set up the chairs, tables and display, but before any participants arrive.

PRACTICAL SUGGESTIONS FOR DELIVERING SESSIONS

Be prepared and read the background topic material. Know the information, but listen to what the participants are saying. Share your own experience, but mostly pick up on themes or stories from the participants.

Asking a well-placed, open-ended question can prompt group members to come up with much of the information themselves. You can follow up with relevant information, then clarify the messages and add further information.

The fall and safety stories

Refer, once again, to the 'Background' chapter and the section: 'Storytelling – using stories to facilitate learning and develop confidence'. This section will prepare you to be able to listen to people's stories and their meanings. With such preparation and with practice, the facilitator can (using the group process) help the participants overcome barriers, assist them in reframing negative thoughts, and support them in making changes that will keep them safe. The 'Background' chapter is essential training.

Repeating common themes

There are a number of connected themes that recur throughout the program. These themes are key concepts and arise from applying our current knowledge of falls prevention in response to the common issues raised by participants across programs. Repetition by the facilitator can give special emphasis to such key themes.

These themes include:

- It is not inevitable that you will fall more often as you get older.
- When out walking, scan ahead to be aware of hazards, and walk heel-and-toe while scanning ahead. There are many potential causes of a fall, and you can become much better informed about these factors.
- With knowledge, you can be in control of falls.
- One of the main reasons you lose some of your balance reactions as you grow older is that you are not testing them constantly. Challenge your balance and it will improve. Keep doing it and you won't lose it.
- Once you lose your confidence due to falling, you may start to limit your lifestyle. This can be redeemed with knowledge.
- Both older and younger people can have falls. It's just that when we are older, the chances of an injury are greater.
- You can gain strength in your legs very quickly at all ages.
- Better balance and stronger leg muscles will protect against falls.
- Become aware of wet, slippery surfaces and other obstacles.
- Remember to lift your feet up off the ground and walk heel-toe, scanning ahead for hazards when walking.
- As your strength and balance improve, walking will become easier.
- If you are someone who rushes, slow down your pace a little.
- Don't give up; maintain your gains – an insurance policy for independence.
- Now is the time to look after yourself.
- Falls are not inevitable.

Remember, don't look at your feet. Scan ahead so you can see obstacles in your way.

The program seeks to increase the confidence of participants in their ability to keep themselves safe, and to validate them as worthwhile citizens with many productive years ahead. Negativity is avoided. A positive attitude is vital.

Using prompts to stimulate discussion

We have simplified the Janis and Mann[1] decision-making process and reframed it into the following list of questions. These questions are used as a basis for discussions about preventing falls and for encouraging follow-through with safety strategies. They can be used as prompts in response to participants' stories, to encourage thinking and movement through the decision-making process about what can be gleaned from each story.

Preventive framework (for reflecting on fall stories)

1. What are the causes of falls, and what are the consequences?
2. How can you stop falls in the future?
3. How can you make this happen?
4. What are the barriers to you making this happen?
5. How can you keep this going? What are the benefits?

Adapting the framework to stories about safety strategies

1. Why did this work/not work and what are some other things that could work?
2. Which way works best for you?
3. How can you make this happen?
4. Are there any barriers to you making this happen?
5. How can you keep this going? What are the benefits?

These frameworks guide discussions about falls and safety strategies throughout the sessions. Be aware of when participants are moving through the various stages of the framework.

The questions don't always fit within the discourse in the exact way we have presented them. However, as you listen to the participants' stories, think about the framework and how it can be used as a working tool. Choose the prompts to fit the situation.

---

1   Janis & Mann, 1977.

The homework

Homework is given each week, including the need to keep track of weekly exercise. The homework is reviewed at the beginning of every session and encouragement given. We are careful to remember to check the weekly exercise records each week. If participants know they will be asked to give feedback the following week, they are more likely to be committed to following through. The follow-up also acts as a time for reflective learning and an opportunity for clarification.

Remember to ask: What three things do you remember from last week?

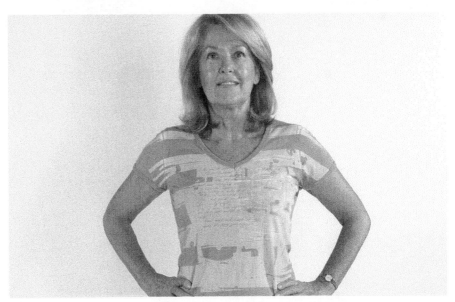

Fun and humour

Having fun and using humour can build group cohesion and a positive learning environment, supporting creative thinking. A well-paced group that has time for fun, sharing relevant comments and stories, and good humour is likely to be an engaged and successful group.

Preparing for each session

The Stepping On facilitator should familiarise themselves with the content in the topic sections and be able to answer questions. This also applies to topics where they have an expert guest. They will need to be able to support the expert in their content area, answer questions and keep the expert on track.

Catherine Vi, past Stepping On facilitator

What I've learned:

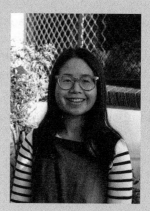

- little strategies such as road safety, medication reviews in the home, and carrying a list of medicines
- recommended daily intake of vitamin D and calcium (especially for the older person)
- specifics on footwear that I was previously unaware of, as often this goes beyond the field of physiotherapy

The good:

- lots of discussion with older people engaged in their learning and becoming empowered in the process
- seeing people changing and improving their quality of life! Very rewarding!

The bad:

- managing the waiting list – especially inappropriate referrals

How it has changed my clinical practice:

- I ensure that I always take a holistic approach to cover all the facets that can contribute to a person's falls risk such as home safety, community/road safety, meds, diet and footwear.

DEBRIEFING

Allow time for the facilitator and co-facilitator to meet briefly at the end of each session. This is essential for ensuring that individual and group needs are met. Reflect on how the session went, any specific issues that arose, and any changes or specific emphasis needed for future sessions.

FURTHER READING

Clemson, L., & Swann-Williams, M. (2010). *Staying power: tips and tools to keep you on your feet*. Sydney, NSW: Sydney University Press.

Hill, K., Clemson, L., & Vrantsidis, F. (2006). Preventing falls – a key to maintaining independence. In H. Mackey & S. Nancarrow (Eds.), *Enabling independence: a guide for rehabilitation workers* (pp. 182–202). London, UK: Blackwell.

Waldron, N., Hill, A., & Barker, A. (2012). Falls prevention in older adults. Assessment and management. *Australian Family Physician, 41*(12), 930–935.

RECRUITMENT BROCHURES

A MS Word version is available from the Sydney University Press website: sydneyuniversitypress.com.au/stepping-on-2019

Session 1
—
Introduction, overview, & risk appraisal

OBJECTIVES

The main objectives of this session are for participants:

1. to build trust so that they feel comfortable to share their knowledge, ideas, questions and answers with one another and with the group facilitators, setting a tone for the rest of the group meetings
2. to understand that others have falls and that there are a variety of reasons why we may fall
3. to recognise the importance of exercise, strength and balance in preventing falls
4. to realise that through this group process, a great deal can be learned from one another.

RESOURCES FOR SESSION 1

Session materials: Session 1 agenda; name tags; attendance sheet; display board and display items; flip chart, butcher's paper or whiteboard; marker pen; door signs; pens for participants to use.

Handouts and flyers: outline of the Stepping On program; 'Balance and strength exercise manual', which includes weekly exercise records; 'Shopping list'.

Catering: snacks and beverages for break.

Other resources: leg weights (demonstration only).

PREPARING THE EXERCISE SPECIALIST

Send a letter to confirm date, time and location, and resources. If the exercise specialist does not already have a manual, provide a copy of their segments and background topics. Send also:

- Session 1 and Session 2 outlines ('Exercise review' and 'Moving about safely' segments)
- At Session 2 provide them with the Session 6 outline ('Mobility mastery' segment)
- 'Balance and strength exercise manual'
- Articles: Clemson, L., Cumming, R. G., Kendig, H., Swann, M., Heard, R., & Taylor, K. (2004). The effectiveness of a community-based program for reducing the incidence of falls among the elderly: a randomized trial. *Journal of American Geriatrics Society*, *52*(9):1487–1494.
- Topic: 'Exercises to protect from falling' including the table 'The exercise benefits, modifications and upgrading: some tips and comments'.

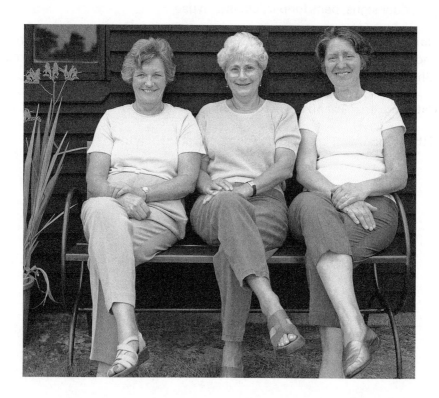

Outline of Session 1: Introduction, overview, and risk appraisal

1.1 INTRODUCTIONS 45–50 MIN	Introduce group facilitators.
	Housekeeping: 'Where are the toilets?'
	Housekeeping: 'Turn your mobile phone off.'
	Break: When and where?
	Ask participants to introduce themselves and explain why they are here.
1.2 SUMMARY OF THE PROGRAM AND AIMS 2 MIN	What we will cover and how the program will run.
1.3 YOUR VIEWS: USING THE SHOPPING LIST 5 MIN	Distribute the shopping lists. Ask participants to tick items they want included in the program and to add any extras.
	'We want to know what you want, so this is your chance to tell us. We can all learn from you. You have a wealth of information and life experiences that can help other people.'
1.4 BALANCE AND STRENGTH EXERCISES 8 MIN	Introduce your guest speaker.
	Example: 'We're lucky to have (*name*) who is an expert physiotherapist (or exercise physiologist). These are the exercises that we know work and we want you to be able to do them.' Briefly explain the benefits from and the reasons for these exercises and demonstrate them.
BREAK 15 MIN	

1.4 BALANCE AND STRENGTH EXERCISES (CONTINUED)
40 MIN

Now practise each exercise, explaining the benefits from and the reasons for each particular exercise as it is taught. Answer any questions. Review the safety precautions.

Mark the section of the exercise log to be done during the next week (see homework).

1.5 FALLS RISK APPRAISAL
5 MIN

If available. Otherwise, share 'falls' stories.

1.6 HOMEWORK
3 MIN

'Think of a fall that you or a friend has had. Consider its possible causes. How might it have been prevented?'

'Practise the strength exercises at home at least three times during the week and the balance exercises daily. Fill out the weekly exercise records in your exercise manual. Bring the exercise manual back next week.'

Ask participants to mark the weekly exercise records to be completed during the next week.

1.1   INTRODUCTIONS AND SHARING CONCERNS AND EXPECTATIONS (45–50 MIN)

Welcome the participants to the program. Introduce yourself and the other staff present, explain why they are here and provide their background.

Do the housekeeping:

- Explain location of the toilets.
- The break is an important part of the session – discuss its timing and the fact that the speakers will be available for questions during the break.
- Point out the display.
- Request that participants inform the facilitator if they are going to be away. Explain that this information will be passed back to the group. (This generates a sense of responsibility and commitment.) Ensure participants know who to call and have their telephone number.
- Ask participants to turn off their mobile phones.

Introductions

Introductions are a very important trust-building exercise. Ask the participants, one by one, to 'Tell us who you are and why you are here.'

This is the first time for many of the participants that they will be sharing with the group their views about the causes and the consequences of the falls they have experienced. It is not easy for many people to talk about their falls, so building trust is essential.

Give ample time to each participant for their personal introduction. Let each person tell their story without interruption, so that they have the sense that what they say is being validated. They will then sense that the group will listen to them in the future. This is the most important first step in building trust. Everyone will want to know about the other participants: who they are, their background and their reason for attending. Nothing is learned until this is worked through.

Positive responses from the facilitator that reflect deeper-level listening are important. If someone has a real fear of falls, or if they are motivated to keep their independence, or just want to improve their balance, acknowledge this. Your comments need simply to reflect what each person says.

Make sure that everyone has an opportunity to speak before moving on to the next part of the session. Be aware if someone is taking too long and tactfully move to the next person.

Asking, 'Why are you here?' may elicit some fall stories, and risk appraisal may commence, without necessarily having to use the alternative exercises below. At this stage, the stories usually are about the causes and the consequences of falls. Very often, participants admit that they have lost their confidence in walking about outdoors. Many mention that their balance is bad. As a result, they often walk looking at their feet and do not enjoy the experience of being out at all.

One lady admitted that the main cause of her falls was her poor eyesight. She was ready in subsequent sessions to look at other reasons and explore alternatives to compensate for her poor vision.

Another participant explained that her falls were caused by limitations in her mobility, and that she had been told to take a walking stick when she went out. The others asked her, 'Well, why don't you?' This was a particularly strong and vocal group, and it was evident from Week 1 that the participants felt comfortable validating, challenging and supporting one another.

The stories reinforce the fact that falling and mobility are important issues. People begin to realise that the reasons for falls can be more varied than they had thought, and that their views and experiences are important and useful.

Remember:

- Listen to everyone, make sure everyone has an opportunity to share a story and be heard – just let it happen.
- Remember adult learning principles. Listen to the participants and respect their views: they have considerable experience, and they are experts. Peer support is important, and participants will learn from one another because the group process is happening.
- Thank people for their contributions. Make comments that are affirmative and reflect listening, such as: 'So you value your independence.' 'You can do some things, but you hope to improve your balance.' 'You would like to be able to walk with more confidence.' 'You have really lost your confidence since the fall.' 'That's great; you've come to the right place.'
- Read: 'Storytelling – using stories to facilitate learning and develop confidence' in the 'Background' chapter, which helps with how to deliver this segment and how to deal with storytelling throughout the program.

- Make notes on your attendance sheet after the session about the participants' beliefs about causes of falls and the kinds of issues that were raised. These notes will help you in listening to individual needs and in planning the content for future sessions.

Alternative suggestion: If the group is having difficulty in talking about their falls, it is helpful for the facilitator to begin by describing a personal fall experience of their own (we have all had one). Mention that when worried about falling you tend to shuffle so it is important to start to practise scanning ahead for obstacles in the way rather than looking down at your feet and concentrate on heel-toe walking as you get stronger. Even though the consequences from a fall can be quite different for a younger person, this will be an encouragement to others to begin to talk.

1.2 SUMMARY OF THE PROGRAM AND AIMS (2 MIN)

(Hand out the Stepping On program outline)

Briefly introduce what will be covered and how the program will run. Give an outline of the major topics to be covered. Give recognition to the fact that the participants already have some knowledge about falls prevention and that they will bring this to the group. Mention that the program will cover strategies that have worked in international research studies on interventions to reduce falls.

Five of the major areas are:

1. exercise, balance and mobility (moving around safely)
2. home fall hazards and safety strategies
3. medication review and management
4. footwear
5. vision.

'The program will cover other areas that have also been proven to reduce falls. It will also cover the kinds of things *you* think may cause falls, as there are multiple risk factors for falls. We want to find out what is relevant to your circumstances and to include in the program things you may feel you need to cover.'

1.3   YOUR VIEWS: USING THE 'SHOPPING LIST' (5 MIN)

(Hand out the 'Shopping list')

This exercise is designed to find out the kinds of issues that the participants feel are important to them. The feedback will be used to fine-tune session planning.

'We're going to use the "Shopping list" to create a list of topics we can cover. First, we'll ask you for your ideas, and then we'll provide a list to help prompt you further. We will then spend some time "shopping" to find out which ones you actually want to "buy" and include in the program. We can revise this at any stage.'

Brainstorming activity: 'What topics would you like to see covered in this class?'

Hand out pens and the 'Shopping list' as a way of prompting suggestions. Ask each person to tick the topics they are interested in and to add anything else they want to learn about. Always read the list out for those people who might have literacy or English reading limitations and do not want to disclose this. After the session finishes, the list must be tallied so that it can be presented in Session 2. Participants like to know what kind of issues people are interested in and that you were interested in knowing what they want and which were most popular. Plan to incorporate this list into the program. For example, it might influence the kinds of questions when considering home falls hazards, or the kinds of 'mobility mastery experiences' to be used in the outdoor walk in a later session or the kinds of community resources that might be helpful.

1.4   STRENGTH AND BALANCE EXERCISES (8 MIN INTRODUCTION + 40 MIN)

Introduce the guest speaker, their expertise and how it relates to falls prevention.

Note: We find it less confusing if the PT explains the exercises first and later gives out the exercise manuals.

The guest speaker now shows the group the 'Balance and strength exercise manual' and where the weekly exercise records are in the manual. They introduce the exercises briefly and explain their importance in preventing falls through improving balance and strength. Explain that participants can improve their balance and strength. Unlike our elite athletes who have to train extremely hard to get even small gains, you will be able to feel your legs growing stronger within a couple of weeks.

Explain that there are balance exercises that can be done daily and strength exercises that should be done at least three or four times a week. If they practise, participants will see a difference quite quickly – their legs will strengthen and their balance will improve. 'We will show you how to improve your balance by challenging your balance in some simple ways.' Improving balance is a less familiar concept than strength training, so it is important to emphasise how important it is to fall prevention.

> Combine a practical demonstration of each exercise with clear and simple explanations (see points below and draw on the information in the topic when relevant). Tell them they are going to get a manual but that they should first watch the demonstration, and that the group will then practise together.

Balance exercises (can be done daily and even embedded into some daily routines):

- sideways walking
- heel-and-toe standing
- heel-and-toe (tandem) walking (upgrade only)
- sitting to standing

Strength exercises (at least 3 or 4 days a week):

- knee–strengthening exercises
- side hip–strengthening exercises
- calf raises.

Now hand out the manuals and ask the participants to practise each exercise with the 'Balance and strength exercise manual' open in front of them.

As a cue, the participants record in their manual the number of times they do the exercises. The following points are reinforced as the exercises are introduced. It is helpful for further information to be given while participants are practising the exercises, especially if such information is an answer to participants' questions. Encourage questions at all times, since this gives participants a sense of ownership of the information.

Talk about the benefits of the exercises, avoiding jargon and using physical demonstrations to keep the explanations simple and clear. For example, saying 'The quads, the big muscle here …' makes it clear where the muscle is, and a demonstration can show what it does (see points in the Topic section).

Explain the benefits simply, reminding people, 'This one is for balance,' and 'This one is to make your legs stronger.' The connection between doing the exercises and their actual value begins at this point. Give a clear explanation, with visual demonstration where possible, of how the balance and strength exercises specifically relate to preventing a fall, regaining balance when finding oneself off-balance, and other fall-relevant goals, such as 'heel-and-toeing' when walking. Emphasise the importance of scanning ahead while heel-toe walking.

· ·

'You helped us understand why we had to do these, and why we needed to keep doing them. You didn't just tell us what to do. You listened to us.' – MARY

· ·

Explain that it is important to report a painful back or painful knees, for example, so that the exercises can be adapted. Conveying the idea that the exercises can be adapted for individuals is important in itself.

Limit the number of repetitions at first and progress steadily as gains are made. Hold for a count of five in Week 1 and do each one five times. This gives a reasonable starting place. Make sure that the muscle is relaxed each time in between the repetitions.

Explain that the exercises can be upgraded in different ways (by increasing repetitions, by adding weights for strengthening, and by using no hands to increase the challenge for balance). The guest speaker should assure participants that they can exercise at a pace and level that suits them individually. 'The Stepping On facilitator (name) will help you practise them each week, and also to upgrade them. If you have any problems the facilitator can contact me with any specific questions for modification or tailoring for medical conditions.'

Give permission to 'snack' on exercises if that is helpful. For example, some people will do a few exercises first thing in the morning, and the rest while watching TV later in the day. We find it useful to clarify that participants need to complete one exercise fully in one sitting; for example, using the left leg to do an exercise, then the right leg to do the same exercise needs to happen at the one exercise time.

Mention that walking is also good, and encourage people to walk on a regular basis. Research has shown, however, that walking alone will not prevent falling. In fact, people need to be stronger to walk better. 'If you do these exercises and can keep them up, then you will find that walking is easier and more pleasurable. These exercises are to help you with your balance and strength, and stop you falling when doing all the things you need to do during the day.'

The therapist watches as they practise and adapts accordingly while still maintaining the group process.

Modify or upgrade the exercises for individuals as required. See table 'The exercise benefits, modifications and upgrading: some tips and comments' for detailed suggestions.

Explain that to be really beneficial, strength exercises need to be done at least three times a week, and that balance exercises can be done more often, preferably daily. When done at a regular time, they will become routine or automatic.

Demonstrate the leg weights in Week 1, if appropriate. Usually we wait to Week 2 to give them out, and concentrate on starting the balance exercises in Week 1.

Suggest that it is best for most people to do the exercises for at least one week before using the weights. Upgrading can be done by increasing the number of times the exercises are done and then by introducing and increasing the weights.

The weights will be used with the knee–strengthening exercises, the leg raises, and the side hip–strengthening exercises.

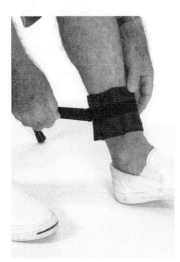

Demonstrate how to put the weights on.

Explain that participants can swap a weight at any time for one that is heavier. This happens throughout the program, and participants will begin to report positive feedback about the benefits of the exercises. For example, 'My balance is better,' or 'My foot drop has improved.'

Have information available about the purchase of the leg weights used in the class demonstration. Bring some examples of homemade leg weights.

For additional information, see the 'Exercise' segment in the 'Topics' chapter and the *Otago exercise programme to prevent falls in older adults* that is listed in the 'Stepping On workshop facilitator supplies' chapter.[1] Both are essential reading.

> We have found that as the group progresses, people start to work out that they have to keep doing these exercises for life. They need to work this out in their own time. Most importantly, we respond very positively whenever someone realises that the exercises actually do link to preventing falls and that they need to do them regularly. We take every opportunity to ensure that they share this realisation with the whole group.

The guest speaker should tell participants that they will be back next week to go through the exercises again and to talk about strategies for 'Moving about safely' and 'Getting up after a fall'. Tell them to bring the Exercise booklet each week.

The guest speaker now hands over to the program facilitator, who will thank them for coming.

1.5   FALLS RISK APPRAISAL (5 MIN)

Tell a fall story from this manual such as Mrs Jardine or Mrs Matthew, or alternatively a fall story of your own about an older person, to facilitate guided discussion.

After telling the story, the discussion is guided by following the preventive framework prompts 1 and 2. 'What do you think could be the causes of a fall in this situation?' and 'What could you do to stop the fall in this situation?' The primary purpose at this stage is to raise awareness, but not necessarily to find all the solutions. We use the preventive framework for reflecting on the fall stories and adding meaning and structure. Some of the responses may reflect that people are able to move on to the later stages: 'Making it happen', 'Exploring barriers', and then 'Keeping it going'.

Read 'Mrs Jardine and the night fall'. Use the preventive framework to prompt discussion. It demonstrates both the physical and emotional consequences of a fall, but can also move the discussion on to finding solutions and barriers.

---

1   University of Otago Medical School, 2003.

MRS JARDINE AND THE NIGHT FALL

This day Mrs Jardine seemed particularly anxious as she ushered in her therapist. She has always felt she enjoys reasonable health, despite a 'bad back' and stiff knees and hips. She notices sometimes she has misplaced things when putting them down near the edges of counters and has blamed this on failing eyesight due to the cataract in one eye.

She has talked of other falls, but these have been of little consequence, except for the time she tripped over the kerb in the local shopping centre. She blamed it on her bifocals. She now prefers to stay at home and is happy surrounded by her treasures in her clean and practical villa, with its little comforts and focal areas oriented around her day and evening activities.

As they walked through to the lounge, Mrs Jardine showed the therapist the large bruises on her leg and her head as she blurted out the events of a few nights ago. She sometimes has to get up at night to go to the bathroom, but is inconsistent about keeping a flashlight near her bed. At times she leaves a night-light on. On the night she had the fall she did neither. She got up in the early hours and needed to go to the bathroom. It was pitch dark and she groped around, and in her haste she could not find the bathroom light. She sat down on what she thought was the toilet and her bladder 'let go'. She moved back on to the 'seat' but, too late, realised she was sitting on the edge of the bath, and she fell very heavily on her back and her head. She said,

> 'I couldn't get out, and my bladder gave away terribly and I soaked myself. I was in shock. I took off my nightie and singlet and was just sitting there in the pitch dark.'

She felt very cold and very frightened, and for a long time she did not think she could get herself out of the bath. When she moved, she realised her back was in pain, and the side of her head was bleeding. She finally managed to wrap the nightgown around the taps and gradually turned over on to her knees.

> 'I then pulled myself up after it seemed ages. I don't know how, but I pulled myself up on the bath and stood there for a moment, then crawled along the edge of the bath. I got the other leg out with the help of the vanity and by this time was drenched. I'd wet myself so many times I was flooded — a horrible feeling.'

At a visit some time later, it seemed the horror of that stressful night still plagued Mrs Jardine. She also talked a lot about her worsening back, and it was evident her mobility had deteriorated. She thought things were 'somehow changed' since the night fall. In some way, her confidence and self-esteem were altered. Mrs Jardine is clearly asking for help and is now fearful of her future.

Brainstorming activity: Mrs Jardine and the night fall

What factors do you think may have contributed to Mrs Jardine's fall?

- no night-light
- feeling urgency
- poor balance
- having cataracts and poor night vision
- lighting behaviour at night: are lights used, and (if so) which lights are used?
- not accepting ageing changes, so does not believe she needs a night-light to help her orientate in the dark
- relies on her memory rather than strategies to automatically switch on a night-light
- Is the light not used at might because it makes her more awake and alert? Instead, should soft way-finding lighting be considered?
- increasing isolation, going out less, and anxiety

Are there any other plausible explanations?

What could she now do to be safer at home and feel more confident?

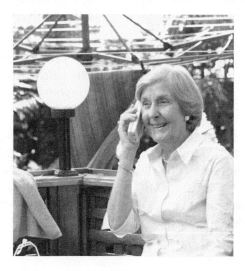

MRS MATTHEW'S FALL IN THE KITCHEN

It seemed a usual sort of day, with Mrs Matthew busy baking her favourite biscuits for the grandchildren who would be sure to visit on their way home from school. She and her devoted husband have chosen as their retirement house a little holiday cottage in a friendly country town. She prides herself on its neat, uncluttered, and very organised appearance.

Mrs Matthew is healthy and spritely, apart from a recent bout of the flu that has been difficult to shake. In fact, it was Mr Matthew, who moves much more slowly than his wife, about whom the occupational therapist had some concern regarding falling, what with the open curved spiral stairs inside and the steep wooden stairs at the back of the house.

Mrs Matthew had just placed the tray in the oven and turned towards the table to put down the oven mitt when it happened. The fall took her by surprise and she was rather concerned for some time after. She found herself going over the events of that day and asking herself: How did that happen? It was so unexpected! Might it happen again? What if it had been Mr Matthew? She felt a chill as she pondered a worse scenario if it had been her husband who fell. He would surely not have recovered so quickly.

Brainstorming activity: Mrs Matthew's fall in the kitchen

What do you think may have caused her fall and what strategies might prevent either Mrs Matthew or her husband falling in the future? Possible replies might be:

- She had been unwell and falls frequently occur at times of temporary illness.
- She could have taken more care.
- She was rushing and not accepting that she must learn to consciously slow down.
- A spill on the floor might have caused the fall.

Can you think of any other plausible explanations?

1.6 HOMEWORK (3 MIN)

The homework is intended as guided practice and reflection. Participants will be selective in what they try out, and while they may not follow through with the suggested homework, it is important to review the homework each week and also to listen for the stories that are offered about other things they have achieved.

Homework:

- Think of a fall that you or a friend has had. Consider its possible causes. How might it have been prevented?
- Practise the strength exercises at home at least three times during the week and the balance exercises daily. Fill out the weekly exercise record. Bring the exercise manual and record back next week.

End the session by enthusiastically outlining the program for the following week: 'Exercise and moving about safely'. Remind participants what they need to bring with them for the next class.

Exercises to protect from falling

In Stepping On we aim to:

- motivate and encourage participants to:
  - understand the reasons why improving balance and lower limb strength can prevent falls
  - understand the benefit of these particular exercises for improving gait and function in everyday activities, as well as for protection from falling
- help participants learn and practise the exercises by breaking them down into simple steps
- upgrade the exercises to support individuals in reaching their personal potential over the seven weeks
- encourage the participants to develop regular lifelong exercise habits.

SAFETY PRECAUTIONS BEFORE STARTING THE PROGRAM

Many of our facilitators request that participants seek permission from their doctor. Encourage participants to ask questions and inform the physiotherapist of possible stressors and limitations. We ask participants to make sure they are medically able to do the exercises and contact their doctor if while exercising they experience dizziness, chest pain or shortness of breath (that is, if they are unable to speak because they are short of breath). Encourage them to ask questions. When first starting we encourage people to have something to hold on to like a bench or table. Safety is important and should be addressed.

People are asked to report any pain, and exercises are modified if necessary. Contraindications to progressive resistive exercise include hernias or if a participant is currently undergoing treatment for joint problems.

Demonstrate how to put on and take off the weights safely, while sitting. Use a kitchen bench or firm chair against a wall when support is needed while doing exercises. Exercises need to begin within the individual's existing capabilities, and safety precautions should be highlighted as the exercises are upgraded. People need to hold on until they feel confident to be challenged at the next level, without the support.

What is the evidence for balance and lower limb strength training preventing falls?

We know exercise needs to be a core component of any multifaceted fall prevention program. The greatest effects from exercise are when the program has a strong balance-challenging component. This has been consistent across several systematic reviews and meta-analyses,[1] which now includes close to 90 randomised trials. The balance activities need to have a moderate or high level of challenge. Strength training to improve the muscle strength of ankles, knees and hips is also recommended. This makes sense, because as balance improves, having stronger muscle power and muscle quality will aid in being able to do more functionally and will improve gait, stair-climbing, etc.[2]

The 'dose' of exercise is also an important aspect to consider. The exercises need to be done consistently and for at least three hours per week.[3]

Walking alone, as a single intervention, can *increase* the risk of falls, particularly if brisk walking is advised. However, increased walking and physical activity have been safely included in successful trials and should be encouraged *as gait and muscle strength improve*.

Successful exercise programs to reduce falls have been both home- and group-based. Examples of home-based programs include the Otago strength and balance exercise program[4] and the Lifestyle-integrated Functional Exercise program (LiFE), in which older people were taught to incorporate simple balance and strength activities into daily activities.[5] Tai Chi has also proven to be effective,[6] as shown in a systematic review[7] suggesting a benefit of the older Yang style over the Sun style, with Yang tending to be more demanding and performed with a lower stance.[8]

Although in Stepping On we teach some simple balance and lower limb strength exercises to be done at home, people may wish to follow up

---

1   Gillespie, Robertson, et al., 2012; Sherrington, Tiedemann, et al., 2011;
     Sherrington et al., 2016.
2   American College of Sports Medicine, Chodzko-Zajko, et al., 2009.
3   Sherrington, Michaleff, et al., 2016.
4   Campbell, Robertson, et al., 1997.
5   Clemson, Fiatarone Singh, et al., 2012.
6   Voukelatos, Cumming, et al., 2007.
7   Huang, Feng, et al., 2017.
8   Lam, 2017.

post–Stepping On and supplement their home-based exercises with other options or a group program that they know will provide protection from falls. There are suggestions later in the manual for including information here about suitable local community programs.

What is balance?

Balance is the ability to keep an upright posture and keep the body within the base of support and with minimal postural sway.[9] Maintaining balance requires motor planning and the integration of input from multiple sensory systems – vision, proprioception (touch) and vestibular (body movement and spatial awareness).[10] The integration of these systems occurs in the cerebellum, the cerebral cortex and the brainstem, and results in motor, vestibular and ocular outputs to maintain and adjust balance. The way these systems function and integrate can be enhanced by balance practice. Balance is taken for granted, and the fact that it can be improved is not well understood. Once people understand that balance can be improved – and how it relates to function, falls protection and maintaining independence – they can then see the benefit of doing these exercises.

How to challenge balance

Improving balance[11] involves undertaking progressively more difficult activities that challenge balance to a moderate or high degree. The level of challenge needed is individual and should be upgraded as improvement occurs.

Challenging balance needs postural change and weight transfer. The heel-and-toe standing exercise, for example, is excellent for this for many older people, when done correctly. Capabilities are very individual, and this exercise was often challenging to the younger staff as well. Gradually reduce hand support as soon as the exercise ceases to be a challenge and can be done safely without support. The balance benefit becomes evident when hand support is reduced or removed. Isolating from sensory input, such as closing the eyes, would only be done at a very advanced stage.

Ways to progress balance challenges include:

- reducing hand support
- broad to narrow base of support
- wide base to narrow stance, or double-leg to single-leg stance
- doing a functional task at the same time (e.g. tandem

---

9   Shumway-Cook & Woollacott, 2001.
10 Vestibular Disorders Association, 2008 – see figure 1 on the website.
11 Fiatarone Singh, 2000; Sherrington, Tiedemann, et al., 2011.

stand preparing vegetables or while talking on the phone)
- move over the centre of mass (or gravity) – control the body position while standing or walking, e.g. transfer the body weight from one leg to another, sidestep, or reach safely
- involve muscle groups that are important to posture, such as the calf muscles. Thus, calf raises also help with balance
- eyes open to eyes closed.

'If you don't use it, you lose it' applies equally to balance as it does to strength. Balance can be improved and the gains maintained by regular practice. There is very strong evidence that doing challenging balance activities greatly reduces the risk of falling.

Strength training with leg weights

The leg weights are weights that can easily be put around the ankles and secured with Velcro tapes when doing the knee–strengthening and side hip–strengthening exercises. They sometimes have a pouch so that weights can be upgraded. They can be purchased from sports stores or online, or be homemade. You may be able to get a local business to donate payment for them – even if it is just to have some on display each week – or subsidise their cost. Just make sure that the weighting is commensurate with the participants' abilities. Weights should start light and be built up slowly. Leg weights can be introduced in Week 1; however, we prefer participants only start to use them in Week 2, when they are more familiar with the exercises and their own capacities. There is strong evidence that lifting weights of 1–3 kilograms (2–6 pounds) and even more is attainable for older people. We found that in the group situation it was better to start with 0.5 kilograms (1 pound) and upgrade to 0.8 kilograms (1.75 pounds) to ensure that people did not overdo it in the initial stages. We had 1 kilogram (2 pound) and 2 kilogram (4 pound) weights ready for when people were ready to upgrade. Most effect starts at about 1 kilogram. If you are not able to provide weights, then participants need to be supported with information on where to obtain their weights and which type and size. Some participants have made their own weights from rice or sand in a sock or stocking. We have found, in follow-up interviews with people attending community groups, that procuring weights is a major barrier to ongoing home exercises. It is very worthwhile following up in future groups whether anyone is having difficulty acquiring their ankle cuff weights.

PROCESS AND BENEFITS
OF GAINING STRENGTH

Muscle fibre, and thereby strength, begins to decrease after the age of 30, and decreases more rapidly after the age of 70.[12] This can be associated with a general reduction in physical activity. However, weakness and disuse are reversible at all ages. People in their 90s can increase muscle strength by progressive strength training.[13] In fact, older people in particular have a great capacity to increase muscle strength, and this fact can be used in a way that can motivate. It does not take long to increase strength. Older people can see a difference in one or two weeks, and in six weeks can increase their muscle bulk.

A weak, shuffling gait is a falls risk. Strength training increases muscle mass, and therefore strength, and improves bone density. Increased strength of quadriceps has a direct relationship to gait[14] and gives both speed and ability to use the 'heel-and-toe' action with confidence. Weight-bearing exercise reduces the risk of osteoporosis.

Muscle must be overloaded to make any strength gain, and the overload must be progressively upgraded by adding resistance. Gravity may be enough at first. Moving and lifting slowly, avoiding the use of momentum, also adds resistance. Standing up from a chair is a challenging exercise because it is difficult to do in a controlled slow movement. Pausing between each lift allows the muscles to come to rest and ensures that new energy, and not stored energy, is used. Observe how people do each exercise to ensure that they are targeting the correct muscle group.

Progressive resistive training is upgraded by increasing the number of repetitions and by increasing the weight. One set is usually about 5–10 repetitions. Once someone has reached one set they can increase to a second set. 'Progressive' means upgrading slowly and continuously. In the group setting, individuals do this by self-monitoring. The time to upgrade is when they find the exercise no longer difficult to do. Participants should increase weights at various times over the seven weeks, and we encourage this even up to the three-month booster group. To gain health benefits, muscle-strengthening activities need to be performed somewhere in the 'hard to do' range.

A common strength measure is one repetition maximum (1RM): that is, the largest weight that can be lifted through the full range of the motion

---

12   Mazzeo, Cavanagh, et al., 1998.
13   Fiatarone, Marks, et al., 1990.
14   Fiatarone-Singh, 2000.

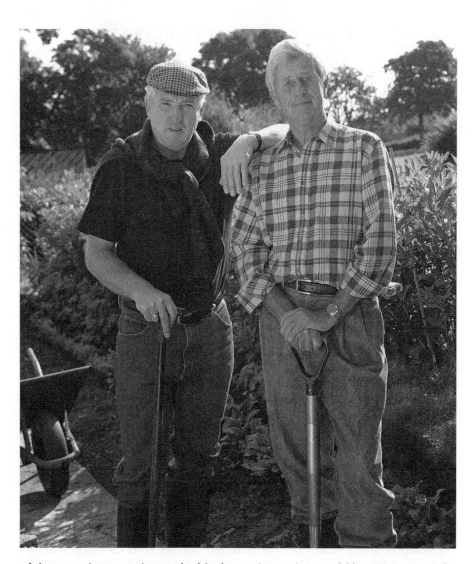

of the exercise, one time only. Moderate intensity would be using a weight that is 60–70 per cent of the 1RM. This is the goal in Stepping On. We do not teach people this directly, however, but start off with everyone using gravity as the resistance for the first week, then we distribute the weights. Standing and exercising with weights will be a challenge for some people, and conducting the exercises where they can hold on for support and correcting their technique is important. We teach participants to take control and self-monitor and to increase weights so they keep working in the 'hard' range.

Walking and being physically active

Strength training improves walking endurance.[15] Strength and balance exercises should be a precursor to aerobic exercise such as walking, although most people do not see this as a natural transition. We have found that improved strength and balance makes walking easier, more pleasant, and safer. Participants tell us they are 'heel-and-toe walking' rather than shuffling and incorporating the safety strategies in the community safety session, such as scanning ahead for hazards rather than looking down at their feet as they walk.

Enabling uptake of exercises

There are a wide variety of barriers to starting and sustaining exercise. The review by Franco et al.[16] found that many older people still believe that physical activity is unnecessary, risky or even potentially harmful. Others recognise the benefits for improving physical and mental wellbeing, but report a range of barriers to physical activity participation. These can be: acceptance of weakness and poor balance as just part of ageing, not enough time, not understanding the need to do exercise or how to do it, fear of falling, lack of confidence in one's ability, lack of a planned program with gradual increases, concerns about pain, discomfort or falling, or lack of immediate physiological feedback as levels plateau.[17]

We address these barriers in many ways in the program, assisting people through the decision-making process to try to reach an ongoing commitment to exercise, and teaching them how to do the exercises and why it is important to do them. Increased knowledge and skill, and a sense of empowerment that they can do them, will make a difference.[18] For example, 'not having enough time' to exercise needs to be reframed as 'how can you fit it into your daily routines and lifestyle?'

Older people exercise to compensate for biological ageing changes, to reverse the effects of muscles being weakened by disuse, to cope with chronic disability or disease, to improve mobility and function, for aesthetic reasons, and for a general sense of wellbeing. Exercise to prevent falls is motivated by the threat of injury and loss of independence. Older people are often motivated to exercise to continue living at home. People's perception that they can do the exercises, and past experience of exercise, are strong predictors of following through with falls prevention exercises.[19]

---

15   Ades, Ballor, et al., 1996.
16   Franco, Tong, et al., 2015.
17   Franco, Tong, et al., 2015; Rosenkranz, Kolt, et al., 2013.
18   Lachman, Jette, et al., 1997.
19   Haines, Hill, et al., 2016.

We all need reminders about how to do an exercise – and of the benefits. Instructions will not all be taken in at once. We help reinforce and answer many questions over the seven weeks.

These are some of the motivators and enablers to exercise (refer also to the 'Background' section about follow-through and habit formation):

- positive encouragement, and understanding the benefits and relevance of the exercises[20]
- knowing how to form new habits and the role of intent, planning, cues and reminders to prompt action[21]
- using cues as prompts to action, e.g. exercise manual left somewhere strategic, exercise fridge magnet
- facilitators being aware of those who are struggling and why this might be
- self-monitoring
- being enabled to exercise, e.g. shown how to put on the weights and where to get them.

We have long known that routine self-monitoring can increase exercise activity by about 35 per cent.[22] The weekly exercise records are checked each week as participants collect their name tags. The facilitator can provide positive feedback when checking them. This is one way of enabling self-monitoring and helping people to get into the habit of regular exercise.

Having a cue for prompting exercise is essential for everyone. Leaving the weights and/or the exercise manual in a particular spot is a cue for exercise that often works.

In our experience, those people who become committed to the exercises find a particular place and time of the day when they can incorporate them into their daily routine. As one gentleman said, 'It's just like cleaning my teeth.' Others may supplement this during the rest of the day, or find it possible to incorporate some of the exercises as they go about their daily life, for example, doing the calf raises or heel-and-toe standing while on the telephone or waiting in line with the shopping cart, sideways walking down the hall or to the front door, or doing the leg strengthening while watching TV at night. A study of the LiFE program showed that by embedding balance and strength training into daily life activities, older people could significantly reduce falls and improve function.[23]

---

20 Franco, Tong, et al., 2015.
21 Clemson & Munro, 2016.
22 Hillsdon, Thorogood, et al., 1995.
23 Clemson, Fiatarone Singh, et al., 2012.·

Targeting the behaviour for change means knowing what the barriers are to action. Find out whether the participants have been able to procure the ankle cuff weights. Do they need help in doing this? How have others in the group done this? Did they use the suggested resources or find something else? Demonstrate homemade ankle weights.

Coping with relapse

Once habits have been established, the most common barrier is a relapse, i.e. not starting again after a break. Maintaining the exercises in a very modified form during illness or holiday periods has helped some people get back to the full routine. It seems easier to increase the amount than to begin again after stopping completely. The three-month booster session gives an opportunity for people to hear how others have coped or struggled with relapses, and gives them a boost to keep going.

Doing balance and strength exercises for life

Exercise has to be ongoing to provide lasting protection from falling.[24] When someone announces they have decided, 'I have to keep doing these!' it is a great opportunity to be positive and affirming. These people can act as role models to others in the group. Don't miss the opportunity to enable them to share this 'light bulb' moment.

In the long term, people may have a preference for either group- or home-based exercises, or may benefit from doing both.[25] In Week 6, we will cover some options to follow up post–Stepping On, and the resources table should include suitable local options. People who have a partner may be more likely to engage in home-based exercises,[26] whereas some people choose group-based exercises for the social contact and sense of belonging, and others may avoid groups because they lack confidence in social situations.[27] Whatever the reason, people need options to maximise the long-term sustainability of their exercise and to increase their potential for upgrading in the future. Further, exercise knowledge and health professional advice is an important determinant of engagement in falls prevention exercises.[28] We aim for our participants by Week 7 to have the skills and knowledge to continue exercising and to be able to discern what features of future exercise programs or groups would be beneficial.

---

24 Sherrington, Tiedemann, et al., 2011.
25 Haines, Hill, et al., 2016.
26 Haines, Hill, et al., 2016; Mahoney, Shea, et al., 2007.
27 de Groot & Fagerström, 2011; Franco, Tong, et al., 2015; Robins, Hill, et al., 2016.
28 de Groot & Fagerström, 2011; Robins, Hill, et al., 2016; Rosenkranz, Kolt, et al., 2013.

Advancing exercise

Challenging yourself with the exercises is key to getting stronger and achieving better balance. Overall, balance exercises are more effective than strength exercises in reducing falls. Strength exercises improve function and help to decrease falls when done in addition to balance exercises.

BALANCE EXERCISES

For balance exercises, the key to advancing is to allow the participant to feel a challenge to their balance. Many studies have shown that people need to continually challenge their balance to decrease their falls risk, and this can show effects quite quickly. It just needs to be maintained. They must continually make the exercise more challenging.

To improve balance when standing, participants need to do exercises standing up, not seated. Numerous studies have shown that older adults with problems with balance can safely perform and progress their balance exercises, whether they do them in a group or at home on their own.

Another key to improving balance is to perform the exercises frequently enough each week and to sustain the exercises over time.

STRENGTH EXERCISES

For people to progress through the strength exercises and become stronger, they must make the exercise more challenging. Their strength may start improving within a week or two and will continue to improve for up to six months or beyond if they keep increasing the number of kilograms on their weights. To follow the guidelines of the American Heart Association and the American College of Sports Medicine,[29] people should increase the weight that is lifted and do enough repetitions to have the sensation of difficulty by the last repetition (typically doing about 10 repetitions, adjusting the weight up gradually so that the tenth repetition is a little tough). This is considered moderate, safe strength training and has been shown to have positive benefits in terms of function for older adults. A moderate-intensity approach has less risk of injury and improved follow-through by older adults. Progressing in a gradual way has been shown to minimise the risk of injury and provide positive reinforcement for small achievements. However, participants should add weights only to the knee- and side hip–strengthening exercises.

For heel raises, they will progress to 20 repetitions to increase the challenge and then switch to using this as a balance exercise by gradually

29   American College of Sports Medicine, Chodzko-Zajko, et al., 2009.

decreasing hand support. For the front knee– and side hip–strengthening exercises, people should add weights when 10 repetitions become easy, generally starting with 0.5 to 1 kilogram and increasing the amount of weight by 0.5 kilogram each time the exercise becomes easy.

Why do these particular exercises?

'Why these exercises?' can be answered by connecting specific exercises to coping safely with everyday functional situations, such as regaining control from a trip or near-fall, walking more confidently, avoiding shuffling by heel-and-toe walking, getting up from a chair, and reaching into a cupboard. Exercise is free and there are no side effects!

There is a need to keep the exercises a challenge for the individual. Everyone is different, and while we recommend that everyone start at a low grade, some individuals will need to upgrade quickly and others will take more time. It is important that achievements are celebrated in the group. Some may need modification of particular exercises due to pain or other limitations. The following table describes the exercises we chose, and the way we upgraded and at times modified them. Comments will also help in breaking down the exercises so that people understand how and why to do them.

SESSION 01

TOPIC

Safety considerations

IMPORTANT: Make certain you thoroughly understand all the exercises before using them in sessions. Understanding the proper technique is paramount to avoiding injury. Ensure you can recognise when a participant is in danger of falling or when they are in pain. If either of these is happening, tell them to stop IMMEDIATELY and re-assess the situation, adjusting their exercise to an easier level, or changing to a different exercise altogether.

BALANCE EXERCISES

As these exercises are designed specifically to challenge balance, they hold an inherently higher falls risk. When teaching these techniques to your group, emphasise that they should remain cautious until they have learned the technique. Also, make certain they all understand the exercises, and remind them that they should not be embarrassed to ask for help, or to have something stable to hang on to while they practise. When first teaching these exercises, you should constantly be looking around and ready to render aid to anyone who is struggling.

STRENGTH EXERCISES

As strength exercises specifically put a load on the body to challenge the muscles, they come with a risk of injury. The use of proper technique and the right weight can mitigate this risk. Participants should be using weights that are heavy enough to give a slight burning sensation in the muscle group being worked, but not so much that they experience any pain in their joints, muscles or connective tissue. Signs of overexertion include laboured breathing, strained expressions, grunts or heaving noises. You must be constantly observing for these signs when participants begin these exercises for the first time and whenever they try adding more weight.

The exercise benefits, modifications and upgrading: some tips and comments

BALANCE EXERCISES

EXERCISE: SIDEWAYS WALKING

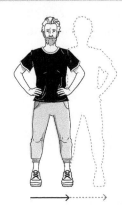

COMMENTS

Do not do too quickly or take too big a sidestep. You can do it, for example, when walking down the hall. Keep your head up. You can hold on to something and then gradually have no support. This exercise is performed facing forward, and with toes facing forward.

TO UPGRADE

- Start with 10 small steps and progress to 10 longer steps (10 to right and 10 to left). Increase repetitions to 10 steps, 4 times.
- Upgrade repetitions.
- Add another set.

EXERCISE: HEEL-AND-TOE STANDING

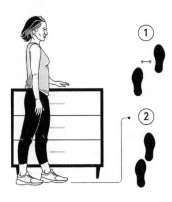

COMMENTS

Tandem standing is an excellent balance exercise. It involves holding balance midway in the stance. It is not about taking steps, but holding balance with one foot in front of the other.

This exercise is often the one people continue to find the most challenging.

Widening the base of support is preferable to holding on. Aim for the experience to be challenging but doable. Progress to tapping the support wall or bench intermittently. Eventually you will stand for longer with no tapping. Alternating weight from one foot to the other, back and forth, is a great way to challenge your balance.

TO MODIFY

Keep feet apart a little, rather than one directly in front of the other. Widen the base of support with your feet.

TO UPGRADE

- Hold position for 10 seconds of tapping.
- Don't hold on.

**EXERCISE: TANDEM (HEEL-AND-TOE) WALKING
                    USE CLINICAL JUDGEMENT**

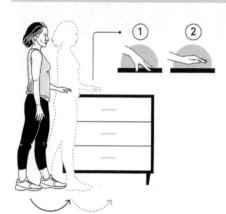

COMMENTS

Tandem walking is a great balance activity. This is an upgrade from heel-and-toe standing. Start in Week 2, based on your clinical judgement.

Move forward slowly by placing one foot in front of the other.

- Increase to 5–10 steps forward.
- Repeat 5–10 steps forward four times.
- Further upgrade to include a tandem walk backwards.

TO UPGRADE

- Start off holding on to a bench, then try fingertip support, then no support.
- Increase the number of times you walk backwards and forwards.
- If you master all these, then try with your eyes closed.

EXERCISE: SIT-TO-STAND

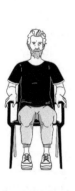 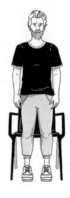

COMMENTS

This should be done slowly to gain maximum strength and to challenge balance. Sitting back down in a slow and controlled manner is also great for challenging balance and improving strength.

The importance of standing up independently can be discussed. However, point out that knees should remain properly aligned and slightly apart while standing and returning to the seated position.

TO MODIFY

Hold on to chair arms.

TO UPGRADE

- Increase repetitions: 5 initially, then upgrade to 10 as usual. To increase further, repeat.
- Go from holding on to chair arms, to holding on to one arm, to not holding on to chair arms, and then crossing your arms. It can also be done from a lower level to improve strength and challenge balance.

STRENGTHENING EXERCISES

EXERCISE: KNEE-STRENGTHENING EXERCISES: LEG RAISES

COMMENTS

This is most important for all our walking, climbing and other activities. Strong knees will help us regain control if we do trip. This is one of the main strength exercises in the program. We can increase our knee strength and our muscle bulk. You do not need to fully extend the knee to get benefit from this exercise. You do not have to fully flex at the ankle either. Doing so will exercise extra muscles, but is not essential. Hold for five seconds, then lower slowly.

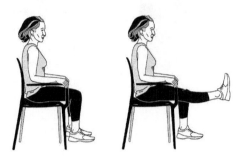

TO MODIFY

This is a good exercise for the knees. You can downgrade it by not bringing your leg up as high and keeping your toes down. If anyone continues to have problems or cannot do this exercise after several weeks, refer for individual therapy consultation.

TO UPGRADE

- Increase repetitions to 10.
- Use ankle cuff weights.
- Increase the weight. Downgrade repetitions.
- Upgrade repetitions.
- Add another set.

EXERCISE: CALF RAISES

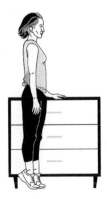

COMMENTS

This combines strengthening ankles and balance. It is very important for strength and control in heel-and-toe walking. It strengthens calves to avoid dangerous shuffle walking that easily leads to trips and falls.

TO UPGRADE

- Increase repetitions to 20.
- Reduce hand support.
- Add another set.

EXERCISE: SIDE HIP-STRENGTHENING EXERCISE

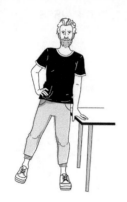

COMMENTS

Another excellent strength exercise. Strong hips means better control and easier walking and climbing, and it is easier to walk over unstable ground such as sand, pebbles or grass. Weak hips have been associated with hip fracture. You need to do this exercise standing upright with the trunk straight. To make it easier, shift your weight onto the weight-bearing leg first. Then, raise leg out to the side. Remember to keep the toes facing forward.

TO MODIFY

People with a back problem can find this troublesome. You can adapt it by eliminating gravity and lying on your back.

Try practising in front of a mirror.

Consider taking a step out to the side in place of lifting the leg out to the side if there is any pain. Demonstration is important.

TO UPGRADE

- Increase repetitions to 10.
- Use ankle cuff weights.
- Increase the weight.
- Add another set.

Key concepts to convey as participants are doing the exercises

Talk about the benefits of the exercises. Avoid jargon and use physical demonstrations to keep the explanations simple and clear. Explain how each exercise prevents falls and improves function.	For example, 'The thigh muscle, the big muscle here,' makes it clear where the muscle is. A demonstration can show what the muscle does. For example, show the thigh muscles engaging to prevent a trip.
Explain the benefits simply, reminding people, 'This one is for balance,' and 'This one is to make your legs stronger.'	The connection between doing the exercises and their actual value begins at this point. Give a clear explanation with a visual demonstration of how the balance and strength exercises specifically relate to preventing a fall and improvement in everyday functional situations. Give examples, such as regaining control from a trip or a loss of balance, walking more confidently, avoiding shuffling by heel-and-toe walking, getting up from a chair, and reaching into a cupboard.

Explain that it is important to report a painful back or knees, for example, so that the exercises can be adapted.	Exercises can and should be adapted for individuals.
	It is important not to overdo it. The concept of 'No pain – no gain' is not true.
	It is okay to feel: achiness or soreness in the muscles for a couple of hours. People may feel stiffness in the muscles after exercise, and even into the next day.
	Delayed onset muscle soreness, where you feel achy, stiff or tight the next day or two, is normal, especially in cases where the muscle has not performed strengthening exercises for a long time.
	It is not okay to feel extreme, sharp or stabbing muscle pain – you need to stop doing the exercise, rest, ice and, if the pain persists, see a doctor.
	To modify the exercises, talk to the therapist in the first and second sessions.
Explain that there are balance exercises they will learn.	For balance exercises, many people need to start with holding on, and that's okay.
	If someone uses a walking stick, he or she should start holding on with both hands. Gradually, people will hold on less and less. This may take several sessions.
	They can start challenging their balance safely (for example, by only having fingertips lightly touching the table or chair) once it's starting to get too easy.
	Get the older person into a safe position with as wide a base of support as possible. They may tap lightly for support. They need to gain confidence in doing the exercises at home, but with a challenge. Correct technique and good posture are important. For example, they should look ahead and not at their feet.

Explain key concepts about the strength exercises.	For strength exercises, start out with a low number of repetitions and increase so they feel they're working a little bit but that it's not too easy.
	It is important for them to have the correct technique at this stage so they target the muscles they are trying to strengthen.
	Hold for a count of five in Week 1 and do each exercise five times. This provides a reasonable starting place.
	Make sure that the muscles are relaxed in between repetitions each time.
	The standing strength exercises start out with holding on with one hand.
Explain that participants can monitor the way they do the exercises at home to make sure they are of good quality, don't cause pain, and don't tire them out too much.	The main idea is that the exercises should feel fairly comfortable, even with the last repetition of the set.
	Participants should not be straining or in pain.
	They should pay attention to how they line themselves up and use hand support so they feel stable and not in danger of falling down.
	They should not get so tired after the exercises that they have to rest a long time or are unable to do their regular activities that day.
	If they are ill or have other significant changes in their life, they may need to modify the exercises and build back up slowly. Remind them that it is okay to miss a day, but they should try to get back into their exercise routine as soon as possible.

SESSION 01

TOPIC

Explain that the exercises can be advanced in different ways.

The facilitator can be flexible about what to discuss regarding advancing in Sessions 1 and 2. For example, the group may include many frail participants. Of course, the facilitator or PT should always answer participants' questions about advancing.

Strength exercises are advanced first by increasing repetitions and then by increasing weights.

Balance exercises are advanced by going to fingertip touching, then to no hands, or doing more challenging manoeuvres.

Assure participants that they can exercise at a pace and level that suits them individually and should advance only when it starts to feel too easy.

Give permission to 'snack' on exercises if that is helpful.

For example, some people will do a few exercises first thing in the morning and the rest while watching TV later in the day.

Clarify that they need to complete one exercise fully at one sitting: for example, all repetitions for the left leg in one exercise and then all repetitions for the right leg in the same exercise.

Explain that, to be really beneficial, strength exercises need to be done at least three times a week on alternate days, and balance exercises daily. When done at a regular time, they will become routine.

Ask participants to fill out the weekly exercise records; this helps to reinforce the exercise routine.

Mention that walking is also good and encourage people to walk on a regular basis.

Research has shown, however, that walking on its own will not prevent falling.

Emphasise that the balance exercises are the most effective in preventing falls – walking should not be a substitute for doing the balance exercises.

In fact, people need to be stronger and improve their balance to walk better.

As they improve the participants have told us that heel-toe-walking and scanning ahead are good strategies to prevent falls and make walking enjoyable again.

RECOMMENDED READING

Franco, M. R., Tong, A., Howard, K., Sherrington, C., Ferreira, P. H., Pinto, R. Z., & Ferreira, M. L. (2015). Older people's perspectives on participation in physical activity: a systematic review and thematic synthesis of qualitative literature. *British Journal of Sports Medicine, 49*(19), 1268–1276. doi: 10.1136/bjsports-2014-094015

University of Otago Medical School (2003). *Otago Exercise Program to prevent falls in older people*. Dunedin, NZ: Department of Medicine and Surgical Sciences, University of Otago Medical School. The Otago Exercise Program is an example of a more intensive home-based exercise program, and it is helpful if the exercise facilitator is familiar with this home-based individually tailored program. www.med.unc.edu/aging/cgec/exercise-program

Session 2
—
Exercise
and moving
about safely

OBJECTIVES

The main objectives for this session are for participants:

1. to recognise for themselves the barriers to and the benefits of regular exercise
2. to be able to do all the exercises correctly and to put on the ankle weights
3. to improve techniques for safe standing, transfers, and climbing steps and stairs
4. to understand that there are ways of getting up after a fall
5. to recognise the importance of not panicking after a fall
6. to identify a plan of action that might work if they did fall.

RESOURCES FOR SESSION 2

Session materials: Session 2 agenda; name tags; attendance sheet; display board and display items; flip chart, butcher's paper or whiteboard; marker pen; door signs; pens for participants to use; summary of 'Shopping list' from Session 1.

Handouts and flyers: 'Getting up after a fall'; 'Moving about safely: goal-setting checklists'; 'Walking stick safety'.

Catering: snacks and beverages for break.

Other resources: leg weights.

Outline of Session 2: Exercise and moving about safely

2.1 WELCOME AND OUTLINE 9 MIN	Welcome back and brief outline of today's session.
	Ask the group for three messages they remember from last week.
	Collect exercise books and talk about last week's homework.
2.2 PROS AND CONS OF REGULAR EXERCISE 30 MIN	Brainstorm the pros and cons of regular exercise.

2.3 REVIEW OF EXERCISE HOMEWORK 12 MIN	Ask each person to report on how they did the exercises or the reason they did not do them. Develop goals for the next week: how to incorporate exercises into a daily or weekly routine.
2.4 SHOPPING LIST RESULTS 1 MIN	Review the 'Shopping list' items prioritised by the group.
2.5 GOAL SETTING FOR MOBILITY MASTERY EXPERIENCES 4 MIN	Choose mobility activities to practise in later session using the 'Moving about safely: goal-setting checklist'.
2.6 EXERCISE PRACTICE 10 MIN	Expert leads the group in practising the exercises. Discuss expected stiffness. Upgrade individuals as indicated.
BREAK 15 MIN	
2.7 MOVING ABOUT SAFELY 30 MIN	Demonstrations and practice of safe mobility techniques, e.g. using a walking stick, getting up from chair, using stairs, and managing kerbs (physiotherapist).
2.8 GETTING UP FROM A FALL 10 MIN	How to get up from the floor after a fall. Demonstration and talk-through by group facilitators.
2.9 SAFETY ALARM SYSTEMS 5 MIN	Let the group know how important it is to get help as soon as possible. Discuss different safety alarm systems.
2.10 FALL STORIES 5 MIN	Ask someone to tell a fall story and explore the possible causes.
2.11 HOMEWORK 2 MIN	Keep doing the exercises. Come up with ideas about what things remind you to do the exercises. What cues do you use? Work out the best time and place to do your exercises.

2.1 WELCOME AND OUTLINE (9 MIN)

At the beginning of each session, ask questions and allow the participants to tell you the answers. Start with how, what, where, when and who questions.

Always ask participants for three things that they remember from last week.

Welcome the participants and give a very brief outline of the day's program.

2.2 PROS AND CONS OF REGULAR EXERCISE (30 MIN)

This segment uses a brainstorming exercise to explore the pros and cons of regular exercise. This activity is adapted from Hoyt & Janis.[1] Use a flip chart for the brainstorming process in order to accomplish this exercise.

The purpose of the pros and cons activity is to think about some of the consequences of exercising and to anticipate some of the barriers to exercising. It is useful for helping people fully consider decisions they are making about whether or not to follow through with the exercise program at home. It provides an opportunity both to explore some alternative choices, and to become more aware of the potential positive effects of choosing to exercise. It also highlights some of the difficulties that people may not have considered previously, but are likely to encounter. Highlighting the barriers to exercising raises awareness so that people can recognise them when they encounter them, which can then lead to attempts to overcome them. This activity has been shown to increase exercise adherence.[2]

- Ask participants to brainstorm: What prevents you from doing these exercises?
- Now brainstorm: What are the benefits of these exercises?
- Use the flip chart, butcher's paper or whiteboard and write the ideas down under two headings: 'for' and 'against'.

---

1   Hoyt & Janis, 1982.
2   Hoyt & Janis, 1982.

The following are some points our participants have come up with:

FOR	AGAINST
• Freedom	• Takes time – have to fit an
• Strengthens your legs	extra thing in
• Makes you feel good	• No place to exercise
• Prevents falls	• Don't have the energy
• Doing something for yourself	• Don't remember to do it
• Lubricates joints	• Too busy
• Improves and maintains	• Friends do other things
mobility	• Bad back
• Improves whole body	• Need discipline and
• Better balance, better control	commitment
• Independence	• Boring

Remember: Be accepting of all responses. For example, respond to a 'for' with a comment like, 'Yes, that's an advantage,' and to an 'against' with a comment like, 'Yes, that can be a problem. It's good you're aware of that.' The aim is to list as many good things and as many negative things about exercising as possible. It is the process that is important, i.e. the process of recognising both the positive outcomes and the difficulties of exercise. Putting these things up front helps people to be more aware of what to expect. They are then in a better position to overcome the difficulties and make exercise happen, or at least to be more prepared to consider different ways of tackling the barriers.

- When all the ideas are listed and acknowledged, discuss both the 'for' and 'against' points.
- Briefly introduce: How might we overcome the barriers? Invite participants to reframe the points 'against' as points 'for.' For example, 'I don't have the energy' can be reframed as 'Well, a lot of the time, by doing the exercises you actually get more energy.'
- End with the questions: Who lives independently in their own home/unit? Who wants to stay there?
- Focus on the benefits: Doing these exercises can help you remain independent.
- Ask the participants if they will make a commitment to doing the exercises during the week. Tell them it helps to actually follow through if you say to yourself, 'I will do these exercises on (Monday, Wednesday and Saturday) morning during the week.'[3]

3   Prestwich, Lawton, & Conner, 2003.

2.3 REVIEW OF EXERCISE HOMEWORK (12 MIN)

Check the completed weekly exercise records. Ask each person how they managed the exercises during the previous week. Invite people to share the various formats and times for exercising that are working best for them. Ask about the barriers people have encountered. Discussing the barriers is useful as many of the participants are likely to still be struggling to get started or to keep it going. Ask the participants to share hints about things that cue them into exercising.

- 'Who did their exercises last week? If you did not do them, tell us the reason. If you did, tell us how you did them.'
- Ask each participant to report any difficulty they experienced, because together you may be able to help work out a better way. Our participants are very honest in telling us when they have not done the exercises, a reflection of the trust built during the first week.
- Ask how they fitted the exercises into their weekly routine. When, where and how did they do them? Encourage group discussion for problem-solving if people had difficulties in fitting them into their daily routine. Brainstorm: How do you fit exercise into your daily routine? Helpful solutions will emerge: 'I do them as soon as I get up and then they're done,' or 'I do them on the bed and then move over to sitting on the edge,' or 'I split them up.'
- Introduce the idea of cueing (identify the enabling behaviour), for example, leaving exercise clothes, shoes or weights in a particular place that is easily seen to prompt exercise in the morning; using a particular television program to prompt the exercises; or sticking a note on the fridge or TV. With prompting, participants will volunteer the different ways they cue themselves to remember exercising.

To move people along to an intention to implement the exercises, ask the participants to think:

'I will do the exercises (where – e.g. in the lounge room) *and will use* (what – e.g. the kitchen bench) *for the balance exercise* (when – e.g. after breakfast on Tuesday, Thursday and Saturday).'

Ask people to mentally make a commitment and say that it will also be homework to write down their 'intention'. Visualising how, when and where is known to help us follow through and prompt us to remember.

2.4   REVIEW THE 'SHOPPING LIST' RESULTS (1 MIN)

Provide the results of the 'Shopping list' tally and outline how the program will reflect their requests. 'This is what we'll cover because you asked for it.'

Ask if there are any further requests for change. 'We will be able to cover all these things over the following weeks. Do let us know if you want more of something or want anything revised or expanded at any stage.'

2.5   GOAL SETTING FOR MOBILITY MASTERY EXPERIENCES (4 MIN)

(Hand out the 'Moving about safely: goal-setting checklist'.)

Moving about safely: goal-setting checklist

Crossing a road	Walking outside	Around the garden
Climbing a kerb	Shopping	What else?
Walking up a slope	Catching bus/train/taxi	
Different surfaces	Walking around the house	

This segment uses the 'Moving about safely: goal-setting checklist' to check where participants lack confidence or would like to improve their mobility. A summary of the group's responses is used to plan the mobility mastery experiences for Session 6. Additional items might include steps, stairs, kerbs, ramps, and lifting/carrying. Remind participants that there is a 'What else?' category.

Add to the list over the next few sessions as stories and issues emerge from the participants.

Begin planning a suitable place now for the mobility mastery experience in Session 6. You may have to book transportation or investigate local parks or shopping areas if no area near your venue is suitable for the needs of the group.

2.6 PRACTISING THE EXERCISES (10 MIN)

(Our guest speaker will complete this section.)

Everyone (including facilitators) practises all the exercises. Each exercise is carefully explained, including the reasons for doing it, which are given while everyone goes through the routine. The therapist corrects any mistakes and talks through any problems or queries. Any aches or pains are confirmed as acceptable or are checked out.

NOTE: If using weights, make sure that everyone understands how to put on the weights. Practise putting them on and taking them off, and make sure the participants can manage the Velcro and fastenings. Weights can be handmade with packets of rice and large socks. As a way of cueing, we highlight in the handouts the exercises that need the weights. Weights are exchanged and upgraded if desired. For some people it is an achievement to graduate to another weight. For others it is an achievement just to try a weight.

2.7 MOVING ABOUT SAFELY: MOBILITY AND TRANSFERS (30 MIN)

(Hand out the 'Walking stick safety' handouts.)

The therapist demonstrates the steps involved and discusses:

- how to get up from a chair
- the correct and safe use of a walking stick
- care of your walking stick – height and stoppers
- the correct and safe use of other mobility aids if relevant to the individuals in the group

- safely climbing steps and stairs
- negotiating kerbs and gutters, using a wider-based gait for stability
- compensating by holding on to things like signposts to assist in negotiating kerbs; learning to scan for useful street furniture
- for those with a stronger leg, encourage them to climb steps, stairs and kerbs by using the stronger leg up/weaker leg down strategy
- scanning ahead.

> The theme is Stepping On safely: walking safely, not shuffling, learning to heel-and-toe walk and scanning ahead, which gives time to prepare for hazards and changes in levels. These techniques are supplemented by the balance and strength exercises. Knowing what to do and having the strength and balance to do it gives confidence.

Gladys from Glebe often used to fall. She told us that she was the only one on the bus one day recently, and the driver recognised her as a regular passenger. She told him she was going to the falls program and showed him the side hip–strengthening exercise holding on to the rail in the bus when it stopped. She loved her new-found fitness and confidence in getting out and about on public transport. She was determined not to be dependent on her family.

Break down actions, such as getting up from a chair, into simple steps and demonstrate them: moving forward in the chair, putting feet together and under the chair, keeping head up, pushing up with both arms if necessary, while leaning forward, and pausing to regain balance before moving.

For people who have one leg stronger than the other, we teach: 'The good go to heaven and the bad to hell,' to help remember which way to step up and down the steps. Although a controversial expression, it is an appreciated and commonly used cue. A walking stick is held on the stronger side and, when walking or climbing steps, moves forward at the same time as the affected leg.

Mention that if they are scared in a crowd to widen their legs, because this will give them better balance on an uneven surface and they will feel more stable.

2.8 GETTING UP FROM A FALL (10 MIN)

Ask: Who has had a fall? How did you get up? What did you do? What system do you have in place to alert somebody?

The aim is to acknowledge how scary it can be – older people worry that they will not be found – and to relieve them of the anxiety by offering coping mechanisms.

(Hand out the 'Getting up after a fall' handouts.)

Getting up after a fall can be a worry for many people. However, group facilitators will demonstrate and talk through the technique of 'How to get up from the floor after a fall'. The following is the method we teach, breaking the process down into simple steps. Use the overhead to present it to the participants as a simple eight-step process. The following explains the steps in more detail so that the facilitator can demonstrate it accurately:

1. Remain calm, try not to panic, and take your time. (What you have feared has just happened, so just stop and take stock.)
2. Bend your knees. (This is a most important step – hips need to be at 90 degrees.)
3. Roll onto your side.
4. Place the upper free hand flat on the ground and come up onto the other elbow.
5. Move onto a fully extended arm and now into a side-sitting position.
6. From side-sitting, come up onto hands and knees so you are into a four-point kneel. Get your balance.
7. Crawl to a chair and place your hands on the seat. Flex up one leg ready to stand. (Alternatively, crawl to the telephone placed in a convenient low place.)
8. Stand up and sit on the chair.

We demonstrate the process, asking the participants to instruct us in the process by talking us through the steps. Alternatively, the co-facilitator will demonstrate as the facilitator talks them through the steps. We also find that people tell us whether or not it worked for them, following a fall. The 'Getting up after a fall' routine gives people time to calm down and a focus on something at least to try, starting with: 'Remain calm, try not to panic, and take your time.'

Discuss other ways to get up off the floor. For example:

- If a knee problem stops you crawling, still use the above method but roll onto your bottom and do a 'bottom crawl'.
- Crawl to a chair.
- Use steps/stairs and pull up onto the step backwards.
- Push up from a sitting position with your back against a wall.
- Leave the phone down low so you can get to it more easily.

Participants sometimes mention they fear being hurt by someone who rushes to help and pulls them up. One participant told us how she instructed the stranger who came to her assistance, saying before he could pull her up, 'Can I use you as a piece of furniture rather than you pull me up? Give me your hand.' The method we teach can be used by participants to guide others.

2.9 SAFETY ALARM SYSTEMS (5 MIN)

Let the group understand how important it is to get help as soon as possible. Ring Emergency 000. You can set up an Emergency App on mobile phones to dial emergency services directly, and to give you a choice of police, ambulance or State Emergency Services.

Reassure the participants that the ambulance will decide whether they need to go to hospital or not. If they lie longer than three hours, it is classified as a 'long lie' because the risk of pneumonia, ulcers, etc. increases. In that case, a hospital stay is likely.

Ask for examples of different safety alert systems people use. Some examples from our participants have included:

- Personal alarm systems (monitored and unmonitored; these have a cost to them).
- A telephone placed in a low convenient place. Relocate the wall phone if necessary. Ask a family member to call daily or use the Red Cross Telecross service.
- A sign to neighbours, such as putting the blinds up every morning. If a neighbour sees the blinds are not up by a certain time, they will check in. Alternatively, if you live in an apartment block, just calling out to the neighbours every day may work.
- Carrying a whistle.

If you can't get up on your knees, try shuffling somehow to get to a phone, sit upright if you can, place something warm over your knees. Ring 000.

Thank the guest speaker for sharing their expertise during this section of the class.

2.10 TELLING FALL STORIES HOMEWORK (5 MIN)

The homework from last week included thinking of a fall scenario. Tell one of your own fall stories or ask the group for a fall story. Now ask the group to analyse it, using the preventive framework to help reflect on the story. The aim is to start the reflective process and for people to feel that there are some answers.

Alternative suggestions: Ask for a couple more stories.

2.11 HOMEWORK (2 MIN)

Return the exercise booklets.

- Remind participants to keep doing the exercises.
- Encourage them to come up with ideas about what things remind them to do the exercises.
- Cueing systems can be encouraged by building a routine so that doing the exercises becomes a normal part of daily living. An example of this would be, 'Oh, the *Midday* show is on, it's time to do my exercises.'
- Encourage them to work out the best time and place to do their exercises, and to write down their intention: *I will do the exercises* (where) *on* (which days) *at* (what) *time.*
- The impact of others' achievements cannot be overestimated. Many will be reporting regular exercise, accompanied by growing strength and improvement in balance, giving self-feedback and incentives for them to keep progressing. Some will stand out as role models and encourage others.
- Participants who plan to get weights will need to come up with a plan of how to purchase them.

End the session by letting everyone know about the following week's program, which will include looking at home falls hazards and safe clothing.

Session 3
—
Home falls
hazards

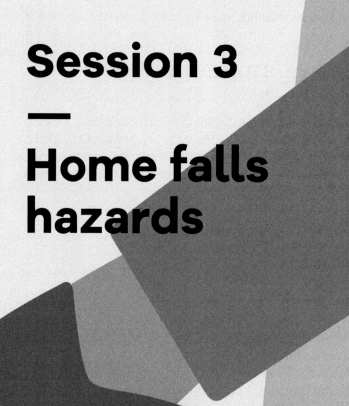

OBJECTIVES

The main objectives for this session are:

1. to raise awareness of the type and range of falls hazards in and about the home
2. to be able to recognise hazards in one's own home
3. to be able to suggest adaptations and find ways to reduce home falls hazards
4. to make some changes at home to reduce the risk of falling.

RESOURCES FOR SESSION 3

Session materials: Session 3 agenda; name tags; attendance sheet; display board and display items (see 'Props' section); flip chart, butcher's paper or whiteboard; marker pen; door signs; pens for participants to use; summary of 'Mobility mastery experiences checklists'; Apple Game quiz; laptop, projector and screen for PowerPoint presentation (if used).

Handouts and flyers: 'Products for slippery surfaces'; 'Westmead Home Safety Assessment'; 'Safe clothing'; 'Safety guidelines when using a ladder'; other relevant community resources and information on community services. An important service is Commonwealth funded MyAgedCare.

Catering: snacks and beverages for break; apples for Apple Game quiz – choose good quality big red apples.

Other resources: leg weights; extension cord; home falls hazard slides or photos, and additional props for display (e.g. slip-resistant products) see 'The display' and 'Stepping On workshop facilitator supplies' chapters.

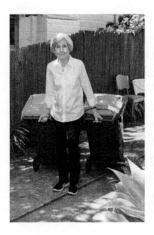 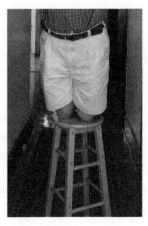 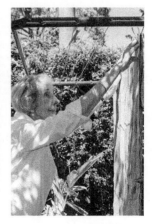

Outline of Session 3: Home falls hazards

3.1 WELCOME AND OUTLINE 4 MIN	Welcome and brief outline of the session. Ask the group for three messages they remember from last week. Review the homework and check the weekly exercise records.
3.2 EXERCISE PRACTICE AND REVIEW 30 MIN	Practise selected exercises, reinforce benefits, and reflect on the cues participants used during the past week. Advance exercises as able. Follow up on the homework.
3.3 APPLE GAME QUIZ 15 MIN	Multiple-choice questions about home falls hazards.
BREAK 15 MIN	
3.4 HOME FALLS HAZARDS 40 MIN	Slides, large charts and props to generate further discussion about home falls hazard solutions. Use a written fall scenario (or critical incident) to prompt discussion using the preventive framework.
3.5 SAFE CLOTHING 8 MIN	Demonstrate hazardous clothing to generate discussion about safe clothing.
3.6 PETS (OPTIONAL) 8 MIN	Ask how many of the participants have a pet. If nobody does, then they may not be interested in this section and you can skip it.
3.7 HOMEWORK 5 MIN	Check for hazards in a room at home or in an outdoors area around the home. Think about what could be changed and report back next session. Keep recording exercises achieved during the week.

3.1   WELCOME AND OUTLINE (4 MIN)

- Give a welcome and briefly outline the session.
- Discuss the homework.
- Did anyone write down their exercise plan?
- When and where did you exercise?
- Check the weekly exercise records.
- What things reminded you to do the exercises each day?
- Listen to the individual achievements and barriers.
- Has anyone had difficulty in procuring the ankle cuff weights?

3.2   EXERCISE PRACTICE AND REVIEW (30 MIN)

Weekly exercise records help to cue some people but not others. Talk about how to 'snack' on the exercises and find out how many times a week people are doing them. Point out that different people use different routines. Two of our facilitators had very different exercise routines, so we provided a good contrast as an example to prompt others to share their differing approaches.

Practise the exercises

Concentrate on the exercises that participants find difficult or have questions about.

When you have the opportunity, reinforce why we do the exercises: 'To stop us shuffling, so we can lift our feet up and move our hips.'

Show the link between the exercises and reasons for doing them, and the gains people are making:

- 'When weaker, our foot moves with the toe closer to the stair tread or is closer to cracks and things we can trip over.'
- 'Ankles get stiff, and that's another reason we trip. That's why we are doing this exercise.'
- 'This one is to strengthen our knees and feet.'
- 'Stepping sideways is for balance. We might be walking or vacuuming; whatever we are doing, we need to have good balance and for our leg muscles to be as strong as possible. It's about strength and balance.'

Advancing the exercises

Why do we need to advance the exercises whenever we can?

Reinforce that people should advance because it increases their strength and balance, which will help functioning and help prevent falls. Regularly advancing exercise is key to preventing falls.

Group members can have the exercise manual open while discussing advancing. For each exercise, point out that the first section discusses general principles on advancing exercises when they become too easy, but each exercise also has specific information on advancing. Encourage people to write notes in the manual on how they will advance each exercise.

The goal is to demonstrate and facilitate a discussion about advancing exercises each week.

> Practise how to advance selected balance and strength exercises.

As you practise each exercise, reinforce good quality posture and movements. There may not be time to practise and discuss how to advance each exercise in this section, so you can spread this over several sessions. The group determines which exercise advances are selected. Find out which exercises people may have already advanced at home. If no one expresses a choice, they can be discussed in the order they appear in the exercise manual.

Advancing the exercises guidelines

Balance exercises. How do people know when they are ready to advance their balance exercises? Each exercise is different; they may advance one before another. Ask people to share how and where they do the exercises so they feel safe when challenging their balance.

Discuss **sit-to-stand**. How many people have increased repetitions to 10? How would you advance this exercise to challenge balance? Ask people to share if they have advanced to not holding on.

Discuss **sideways walking**. How can people advance this exercise to challenge balance? Ask people to share if they have advanced the number or size of the steps.

Discuss **heel-and-toe (tandem) standing** and **heel-and-toe (tandem) walking**. How can they advance these exercises to challenge balance? Ask people to share if they've advanced and how it has gone.

Strengthening exercises. How do people know when they are ready to advance? Ask people to share if they have advanced a strength exercise and, if so, how. Check to see where people are at with the number of repetitions. Are they at the target number of repetitions (10)? How would they know when to add weights? Most people should have reached the target between Weeks 1 and 2. (For some, the therapist may have had to change the target number of repetitions for medical reasons, which is okay.) Many will be using weights. Ask people to share how they put the weights on. Advance the weights for those who are ready, reinforcing that everyone will be exercising at their own level.

Demonstrate how to use two weight bands on one leg for those who need more than two kilograms.

Discuss **front knee–** and **side hip–strengthening** exercises. How can these be advanced?

Discuss **heel raises** next. How could these be advanced?

Practise the exercises, encouraging people to do them at their own level and not to overdo it.

When they get stronger, they can start to let go, using fingertip support for balance; point out that they should start the balance challenge once they have reached 20 repetitions.

3.3   HOME FALLS HAZARDS: THE APPLE GAME QUIZ (15 MIN)

(Have apples for prizes)

The Apple Game quiz is a list of multiple-choice questions about different home falls hazards. This game is a great way to initiate discussion about safety and risk situations, and to identify solutions to these situations. Talk about:

- what people do
- what they could do
- what might be the barriers
- what would make it easier to follow through and do it.

The quiz is adapted from the Apple Game in the *Home safe home: road show*,[1] in which apples are given to symbolise health: 'An apple a day keeps the doctor away.'

---

1   Petch & Smith, 1998.

In Chinese communities, an apple symbolises safety and health and red stands for good luck.

'In this quiz, you choose what you think is the most correct way (or ways) to prevent a fall. The best answer wins an apple.' (We make sure everyone receives an apple. We give out one at the end to those who did not 'win' one.)

For example:

> To answer my phone:
> a) I go as fast as I can in case they hang up.
> b) I carefully check that the route to the phone is free of clutter.
> c) I move slowly and carefully. I leave a window open to hear the phone when I'm outside.
> d) If I don't make it, I don't worry. *They will ring back if it is important or leave a message.*
> e) I ask for a cordless phone for my birthday.

There can be more than one right answer, and discussion flows easily as participants say what they do and what they could do. The telephone question is a good one because people are often not familiar with relatively new products. Those who are familiar can explain, for example, how useful the cordless phone is for them in their situation, what it is and how it works.

You do not have to attempt all of the questions. Be selective. Start the game by choosing questions that relate to the group stories and themes that are emerging. There are more 'Apple Questions' listed in the session's 'Topics' section.

Have the local home handyman service information ready. Do they offer assistance in changing light bulbs? How can people contact them?

3.4 HOME FALLS HAZARDS (40 MIN)

One way to introduce this section is, 'Put your hands up if you have lived in your house five years? 10 years? 15 years? 20 years? 30 years? 40 years? 50 years? 60 years?' Many people have lived in their current house over 30 years. 'Your house hasn't changed much – do you think you have?' A brainstorm exercise on the whiteboard or flip chart:

Some answers:

THEN	NOW
	↓ height
	↓ sight
	↓ balance
	↓ strength

Then ask them, 'If you have had a fall in your own home, where did you fall?'

Use slides, props and fall scenarios to generate solutions.

A slide presentation (or slides printed on A5 cardboard in colour) is used in this section. Hand out the Westmead Home Safety Assessment at the end of the presentation.

Use a slide presentation or colour-printed slides and props to generate further discussion about home falls hazards and solutions. Finish by reading out a written fall scenario for discussion to identify causes and generate solutions.

The slides

The slides have been selected because they reflect the most common hazards found in and around the home.[2] See the 'Topics' section of this session for notes on the 'Home Falls Hazards' slides. Stand at the front near the screen to be able to direct prompts when needed and help keep the group together on the same topic.

Introduce home falls hazards (slide 1). Preventing falls in and about the home could be about:

1. **The place:** Changing the environment (such as putting in a safety rail). 'I had the opportunity of making structural changes to a stairwell in my house. It originally had dark veneer wood walls and was very slippery – I had a fall on it when I first moved in. I put in a skylight and painted the walls a light colour.'

---

2   Clemson, 1997; Clemson, Fitzgerald, & Heard, 1999.

2. **The person:** Changing the way you do things or how you use the environment (slowing down the pace – not rushing, changing how you climb the stairs).

The idea of the slides is to raise awareness of hazards in and about the home. 'We often do not see hazards, such as clutter, because they are part of our everyday environment. They may be a habit that we need to think about, to put into our consciousness for a while so that we can get into new habits.'

The first few slides present some background questions to begin the session and orientate us to the topic (slides 2–8).

The next slides show a list of the most common hazards at home that research has shown are linked to falls:[3]

- slippery surfaces
- obstacles in walkways/clutter
- poor illumination
- floor mats
- footwear
- ladder/stepladder/chair used to climb
- cords on floor
- steps and stairs
- bath
- uneven, broken or loose pathways
- spills on floor
- uneven floor surface.

Question: What time of day do falls mostly occur? Does anyone want to have a guess?

Answer: The graph shows that a peak occurs at 10–11 am in the morning and again in the late afternoon.

Question: Why do you think this may be?

Answer: This is when we are often most active.

Question: Where do falls at home occur? Can someone take a guess?

Answer: The living areas and walkways are the most common place for falls at home. Outdoors falls account for between 20 and 40 per cent, depending on gender and lifestyle.

---

3   Clemson, Fitzgerald, & Heard, 1999.

Slide 12 shows the prompts to use for each hazard slide (slides 13–31), giving a framework that participants can use to a 'pick a hazard' and 'find solutions'. By using the preventive framework prompts, e.g. 'What is the hazard here? Have a look, what's wrong here? What can we do to change that?', the participants are encouraged to make up their own minds as to what the problem is with each of the hazards. Slide 32 finishes with a reminder to participants to apply these questions to their own homes. This leads into the homework.

Props

Pass around the props from the display table as questions and comments arise during the slide presentation. Ask participants to show how the props work or explain how they use them. Encourage participants to provide the answers and give demonstrations. See 'Part 3: Resources'.

Pass other products from the display around and ask if anyone is familiar with them. Discuss how they are used. The display includes poster-size photos, a safe stepladder, a photosensitive light, a lamp, a hands-free telephone, non-slip and rid-moss products, non-slip strips, etc.

The stepladder prompts discussion of when and how to use it. Ask participants to say what the safety features are; the importance of not using the top rung; ease of buying; lightweight and foldable, therefore easy to put away and get out; and ideas about storage. If the ladder is not easily accessible, this becomes a barrier to using it.

A fall scenario

A fall scenario (or critical incident) can be used as a summary of a preventive approach to home falls hazards and gets people thinking. We read Vera's fall[4] to generate a number of possible causes of the fall and then a number of solutions to the problems using the following prompts:

- What factors could have contributed to this fall?
- How might you change that? or How could she do it differently?

The scenarios get people problem-solving and sharing their own stories and solutions. We sometimes use the story of James's fall.[5] The story later in this session outline of the husband and the fall could be also used as a fall scenario. Tell the first paragraph only and then use the prompts as above. The remainder can be added as explanation later, because there

---

4   Clemson, 1997, p. 14.
5   Clemson, 1997, p. 5.

could be many causes (and solutions) generated by this story. Make a note when these stories are used, as after working with a few groups, it is easy to forget which material has been used for whom. The extra ones can be used at a later stage for revision, or as a backup if another session finishes early, or if you just need a change of pace. You might consider using some of the participant stories from Week 1.

....

VERA'S FALL

Vera had just woken up and was feeling a bit groggy from the sleeping tablets she had taken the night before. She shuffled into her old slippers and wandered out of the bedroom. She was feeling light-headed, which made it a bit tricky for her to go down the stairs, but she was thinking more about her breakfast than anything else.

When Vera got to the kitchen, she opened a cupboard above her head and reached up to grab her teapot. The blood rushed from her head and she suddenly felt faint. Vera staggered backwards, trying to regain her balance, but her ill-fitting slippers gave no support and as she stumbled, her feet slid out from under her. She tripped and fell, landing hard on her kitchen floor. Lying on her side in agonising pain, Vera was unable to get up. Then, with final determination, she managed to heave herself up just enough to pull the phone down, and she hastily dialled for an ambulance.

The whole experience was crushing. Apart from the embarrassment, she was in a lot of pain for weeks afterwards because she had fractured her hip bone when she fell. After the fall, Vera's hip never really felt strong again. When Vera finally returned home, she felt intimidated by even the simplest daily tasks. She felt powerless, as though she'd lost control of her life.

....

JAMES AND HIS FALL

James was known in the community for having a busy lifestyle. He was proud of his appearance and loved 'keeping up' with younger people. This 75-year-old had had a number of smaller falls in the past, but he was still very confident about his mobility, always rushing about and having no second thoughts about climbing ladders or running downstairs. It wasn't until Monday morning that the falls became a serious problem. That morning, in his hurry to catch his bus, an uneven piece of the footpath caught James' foot and he tripped. The earth suddenly slipped out from under him and his body plunged headfirst into the gutter. When he fell, he fractured his upper arm close to the shoulder joint. Bleeding and in a state of shock, he was taken off in an ambulance.

During his time in hospital, James cursed that broken concrete, but his thoughts about why the fall happened didn't progress any further than that. It was just an accident, a part of life, so he thought. Then, a few weeks later, he fell again. This time it was a young child suddenly changing direction who made him fall; he saw it as just another accident. And then a few weeks later, he had another fall. It was only after this third fall that James realised he had to think seriously about what was happening.

- What factors could have contributed to Vera's and James' falls?
- What could they have done differently?

Alternative suggestions:

- Use examples from the venue for the program. These are often very visible but not obvious at first to participants. For example, where the cords to the video lie or the safest route to take on the external pathways. At one of our venues, the carpet was looped, so the proprietors had it stretched for us. Programs for young women and children had been held at this venue, but not for older people, and we saw hazards differently. In another venue, the steps had a rail that did not go all the way to the bottom. This prompted talk about safety railings. Use the immediate environment to teach awareness.
- Visualisation game. 'Pick a room at home and visualise the hazards. What can you see? Do this again after the above exercises and see if you notice anything more. Go home and check it. Did you miss anything?'
- Use brief video segments to prompt discussion.

FACILITATORS AND PARTICIPANTS SHARE THEIR STORIES AND SOLUTIONS

'I was in the kitchen and my husband came in from the garden. He was wearing his old RM Williams gardening boots with the worn leather soles. I had been preparing lunches. He was hungry, and it was a hot sunny day. He turned very quickly and fell on the floor. He came down quite heavily on his right side.

'Initially, he thought it was the boots and I thought it was because he was rushing. Later, I realised I had spilled some butter on

the kitchen floor and had wiped it up but had only used paper.
I needed to use a detergent.'

Megan told us a story of how when she was working in her student days in a commercial kitchen, if anyone spilled anything there was a cry of 'Spill!' and no one did anything until it was cleared up.

3.5　SAFE CLOTHING (8 MIN)

(Demonstration of clothing. Hand out 'Safe clothing' handout)

Wear a long-sleeved dressing-gown with ties and big pockets to generate discussion about clothing hazards.

3.6　PETS (8 MIN)

How many of you have a dog? A cat? If nobody does, then they will not be interested in this section and you can skip it.

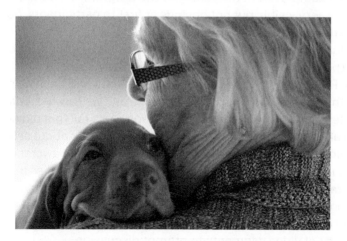

JANE AND HER PET DOG MAX

Jane has a dog, Max, about the size of a cat. Lately, Max had learned to grab his little dog bed in his teeth and move it from room to room.

A very cute pet trick, Jane thought. Recently he started moving it into the front hall.

Before that, the hall had been free of clutter.

One evening at dusk, during a TV commercial break, Jane went through the front hall and upstairs into her kitchen. She noticed the dog bed, with the dog in it, and thought, 'Oh, isn't that cute; he's bringing his dog bed into the front hall!' She did a few chores in the kitchen then was in a hurry to get back to her favourite TV show. Meanwhile dusk had turned to night. She turned off the kitchen light and went into the dark hallway to go downstairs. She didn't notice that it was dark now and she was thinking about the TV show. She didn't turn on the light, and she forgot that the dog's bed was in her path. At the bottom of the stairs, her left foot tripped over the dog in his dog bed and she went down onto her left knee on the floor. Jane didn't bruise or hurt her knee but she felt a sharp pain in the back of her hip, and found she couldn't walk. The force of the impact had travelled up her bone from her knee to her hip, breaking the bone in the back of her hip socket.

Now her dog is at her friend's house, while she is recuperating at home with a broken pelvis.

. . . .

Ask the group: 'What where the causes of that fall? Jane fell over her dog in his dog bed. That's just one way that pets can lead to falls. Let's talk about other ways your pet can put you at risk of a fall.'

Write down people's ideas on white paper or board (e.g. tripping over your pet in the house; tripping over the pet's bed or a pet toy; walking the dog and getting pushed, pulled, nudged, etc.).

Question: What can you do to prevent falling or tripping over your pet in the house?

Answers might include:

- Good lighting
- Colour contrast: if you have a brown dog don't have brown mats on the floor
- Go slow, pay attention
- Obedience school can help your dog learn not to jump on you from joy, and how to sit when told to sit
- Shut the door when you are preparing the pets' food, then walk out to feed the animals
- Put food bowls away from doorways
- Sit on a chair and then put the food on the ground next to the seat so the animals don't run at you
- Know your pet's habits. If he runs up to you at the door, maybe put a chair at the door for you to sit in and pet him when you first get home
- Attach a bell to your pet so you know where it is at all times.

Question: What can you do to prevent falling or tripping over a pet toy or pet bed?

Answers might include:

- Good lighting
- Go slow, pay attention
- Scan ahead
- Use a long handled reacher to pick up and move items out of the path of traffic
- Clean water or food spilled out of the dog bowl right away to prevent a slip.

Question: What can you do to prevent a fall when you're out walking the dog?

Answers might include:

- Obedience school for your pet, so he learns to heel and not lunge at other dogs or cats or amusing telegraph poles
- Make sure you're strong enough to handle your dog if he/she lunges, and if not hire a dog walker (MyAgedCare may be able to help)
- If you can, fence in the yard for your pet
- Only walk your dog in daylight
- Only walk the dog when you think there will be fewer people walking their dogs so they won't get tangled or pull
- Take your dog to a dog park
- Retractable leash (it has pluses and minuses)
- Short leash with tight control (again, pluses and minuses)

3.7 HOMEWORK (5 MIN)

(Hand out 'Products for slippery surfaces' handouts and remind them to complete the weekly exercise records.)

Have participants check for hazards on a walk through their home. They can select a room at home or an outdoors area around the home on which to report back to the group. Think about what could be changed, and be ready to share solutions at the next session.

Enthuse participants for the following week: 'Next week we will explore some very practical and creative strategies for community safety and what we need to know about footwear.'

Home fall hazards

There is strong evidence from meta-analyses and systematic reviews that home safety assessment and environmental and behavioural adaptations can reduce falls.[6] In particular, people who are at higher risk can significantly reduce fall rates by up to 38 per cent. Research supports that it is particularly effective for those who have poor mobility, older people with a history of multiple falls or injurious falls, people with multiple morbidities, those with severe vision impairment and older people recently hospitalised.

The intervention has been effective when conducted by an occupational therapist on a home visit. For an intervention to work, it should:[7]

- identify fall hazards and find solutions, taking into account personal risk, individual capacity, and the person's environment
- use an assessment tool validated for a broad range of potential fall hazards
- actively involve the older person in the assessment – joint problem-solving and ownership of problems and solutions is essential
- suggest adaptations and modifications to reduce fall hazards in and about the home and/or outdoors. The focus is on preventing falls through safety adaptations
- include both environmental and behavioural safety strategies to reduce falls risk
  - Environmental adaptations include raising awareness of potential hazards, removing hazards, adding protective features (such as non-slip stair strips) or assistive devices, adding contrast and improving visibility, moving furnishings, and other strategies to create clear walkways and pathways. Environmental solutions usually do not include major structural changes.
  - Behavioural strategies include using safer behaviours when doing tasks or just when walking around. For example, not rushing to answer a phone, asking for help

6   Clemson, Bundy, et al., 2008; Gillespie, Robertson, et al., 2012.
7   Clemson, Bundy, et al., 2008; Peterson & Clemson, 2008; Pighills, Ballinger, et al., 2016; Vance, Delbaere, & Lord, 2015.

to change a light bulb, regularly sweeping leaves off pathways, using a stepladder safely, or holding the handrail going down steps.

- raise awareness of potential hazards. This also applies to situations such as public places and visiting neighbours, friends and family. Research has shown a visit to the home by an occupational therapist will reduce falls outside the home, even when this was not part of the home intervention[8]
- include adequate follow-up by the health professional and support for adaptations and modifications when needed.

For a full explanation of the occupational therapy home visit intervention to reduce falls, see the Home and Community Safety online training modules at www.fallspreventiononlineworkshops.com.au.

In Stepping On we can utilise many of these key features, enabling the participants to identify hazards relevant to them, share stories of solutions, and learn how to observe their own familiar environments for hazards and plan to make changes. Examples of commonly used items can be on display, along with information on community services for rails or non-slip materials.

HOW FALLS OCCUR

One way of characterising different types of environment-related falls are 'slips', 'trips' (which are disturbances to our base of support) and centre of mass falls (in which we are displaced from our centre of gravity and lose our balance, e.g. by reaching, transferring, bending or turning, sometimes called a 'perturbation').

WHEN AND WHERE DO FALLS OCCUR?

The older people are, the more likely they are to fall within their home, and to fall more frequently. However, there are different patterns of fallers, and in Stepping On we have encountered both: those who fall who are more frail and those who fall who are more active. These types of people are likely to have different risks in different situations.

In a United States study[9] reporting where non-injurious falls occur inside the home, falls were found to occur more frequently in the living areas and the bedroom. Most falls occurred when just negotiating around the home environment or doing everyday tasks. Falls occurred in the bathroom, but this was less often. For injurious falls, bathroom falls were more highly

---

8   Cumming, Thomas, et al., 2001.
9   Stevens, Ehrenreich & Mahoney, 2014.

represented compared with non-injurious falls, but injurious falls in the kitchen and on stairs were also frequent.[10]

Falls and injurious falls can occur at all times of the day and night. But most falls (52 per cent) occur in mid-morning before lunch, or in the late afternoon. These are the times when people are commonly more active.[11]

PROFILING DIFFERENT FALLERS

We can profile people who fall in different circumstances. Those who fall indoors are more likely to be frailer, have a slower gait and poor balance.[12] Those who fall indoors and injure themselves have a particular pattern.[13] The frailer person is more likely to stay at home and falls mostly in the hall and bathroom, very often when visiting the toilet. An analysis of injurious falls treated in emergency departments[14] found 54 per cent were associated with carpets and 46 per cent with rugs. This highlights the importance of considering the transition between carpet (or no-carpet and rugs) to lino or tiles while hurrying to the bathroom. These findings are similar to what is reported in the table below, in which floor mats and floor coverings were identified as a common cause of all environmental falls.

However, there is another group who fall predominantly during activities of daily living. We need to consider fall prevention for healthier and active people, and many Stepping On participants are in this category: wanting to maintain connections with the community, or transitioning to a return to a more active lifestyle following an injurious fall. Those who fall outdoors are more often active vigorous people, doing ten or more activities with a faster gait.[15] Rushing is frequently mentioned as a risk factor, and falls have frequently been attributed to unnoticed balance impairment or deteriorating vision.

Bleiljevens[16] found two patterns of outdoor injurious falls: falls near the home (garden, access paths, climbing ladders), occurring predominantly while carrying out the instrumental activities of daily living (IADLs), and injurious falls away from home, occurring predominantly during walking, grocery shopping or vigorous activity. So home and community safety are both important. First-time falls are often outdoors, so prevention should start as early as possible.

---

10   Stevens, Ehrenreich, & Mahoney, 2014.
11   Day, Kent & Fildes, 1994.
12   Bath & Morgan, 1999; Manty, Heinonen, et al., 2009.
13   Bleijlevens, Diederiks, et al., 2010.
14   Rosen, Mack & Noonan, 2013.
15   Nyman, Ballinger, et al., 2013; O'Loughlin, Robitaille, et al., 1993.
16   Bleiljevens, Diederiks, et al., 2010.

The outdoor injurious fall rates were equivalent in both genders,[17] but the most serious injuries occurred in women.[18] The number of ladder-related injuries from falls is increasing in men over 60 years.[19] It is important to address ladder safety alongside attitude and identity, by recognising risk and changing behaviour.

In interviews with men who had completed Stepping On,[20] we found that the program had challenged them to think differently about themselves and their personal falls risk, and provided practical options for addressing falls risk. They talked about 'adjusting their mindset', by which they meant adopting a more cautious approach, paying greater attention to potential falls risks, being careful, concentrating, slowing down, and 'changing the ways', by which they meant acting purposefully to reduce environmental hazards at home, as well as incorporating the falls prevention exercises into their routines.

TYPES OF HAZARDS ASSOCIATED WITH FALLS

The below table is a summary from a content analysis of studies that report environmental causes of falls[21] completed as part of the validation of the Westmead Home Safety Assessment. The recent update of this review[22] demonstrated these were all still valid, with the addition of snow and ice hazards, which are included in the top category ('slippery surfaces'). Our slide presentation for this session aims to reflect examples of these more frequent hazards, but the discussion needs to be relevant to the group and participants will come up with many other hazards.

17   Duckham, Procter-Gray, et al., 2013.
18   Kelsey, Procter-Gray, et al., 2012.
19   Bradley & Pointer, 2008.
20   Liddle, Lovarini, et al., 2017.
21   Clemson, 1997.
22   Mandelbaum, Clemson, et al., 2019.

Table: Top ten home hazards causing falls

HAZARD	1997	2019	TOTAL
	Clemson review	Mandelbaum, Clemson, et al. review	no. of studies
Slippery surfaces (wet, spills, ice)	41	35	76
Obstacles in walkways/clutter	27	22	49
Ladder/stepladder/ chair used to climb/ distance reaching	12	22	34
Floor mats	15	6	21
Poor illumination	16	4	20
Footwear	14	4	18
Uneven floor surfaces/uneven, broken or loose pathways	9	8	17
Steps, stairs, railing	7	8	15
Cords on floor	7	3	10
Bath	10	0	10

IDENTIFYING RISKY BEHAVIOURS AND ENCOURAGING PROTECTIVE BEHAVIOURS

The following schema to conceptualise behaviours associated with falls is from a content analysis of qualitative studies. This arose from the work developing the Falls Behavioural Scale.[23]

- Cognitive adaptations – behaviours associated with reflection, intention and planning (e.g. taking care when on a new medication or getting new glasses)
- Protective mobility – negotiating the environment in a supportive or protective way (e.g. taking time to adjust one's step when approaching stairs)
- Avoidance – avoidance of risky situations (e.g. getting help cleaning the gutters)
- Awareness and being observant – behaviours associated with noticing hazards and generalising these skills to other situations (e.g. cleaning spills straight away; using detergent on oil or grease spills)
- Pace – slowing down one's pace as a conscious strategy for coping with reduced physical functioning
- Practical strategies – often involve anticipation, for example, using a safe stepladder for climbing, instead of reaching or climbing in unsafe ways.

GENERATING SOLUTIONS

- Using the preventive framework to move into options for change. This can be used to prompt people to find solutions, explore options, identify barriers, and think about how to continue safe behaviours.
- By using a problem-solving approach,[24] our aim is that people will go home and observe their living environment in a fresh new way. This involves brainstorming relevant solutions and weighing up the alternatives.
- Perceiving the risk related to specific situations, autonomy in decision making, and maintaining a sense of control influence the extent to which people will follow through with new safe behaviours.[25]
- It is helpful to encourage people to decide what is the target behavioural or environmental change. What is the action that

---

23　Clemson, Cumming, & Heard, 2003.
24　Gitlin, 2009.
25　Clemson, Cusick, & Fozzard, 1999.

is needed? If the person plans to use a safe stepladder to reach into the top cupboards, how will they get one and where will it be stored so it will be easily used?

- Re-forming habits is challenging, and Lally & Gardner[26] provide a good summary of the considerations involved when changing one's actions in everyday situations:
  - Believe that the change is of benefit
  - Plan and visualise the change
  - Use cues to prompt actions
  - Finally, the targeted behaviour has to be contextually relevant. It needs to be seen to be useful, doable and relevant.

ADHERENCE – PEOPLE DO REMOVE HAZARDS AND SUSTAIN CHANGES

In the original Stepping On trial,[27] we had 70 per cent of program participants adhere to at least 50 per cent of the home falls hazard solutions 14 months after the program finished. These solutions included removing or modifying home falls hazards (e.g. removing clutter, increasing lighting levels, applying non-slip tape to step edges, and fixing pathways). The self-initiated action most commonly reported by the participants at the time of the home visit was the adoption of behaviours associated with community mobility (28 per cent), e.g. heel-and-toe walking and scanning for hazards while walking.

In reality, in successful falls trials of home visit interventions – whether they are exercise or home safety interventions – we consider it a positive effect when uptake one year later is at 40–50 per cent. This requires people to follow through, and for home safety we know this is much more likely if the participants believe it is possible to prevent falls.[28] In the Cumming et al. home safety randomised trial,[29] easy changes such as adding a non-slip mat or moving cords out of walkways had the highest adherence. Using night-lights was often partially adhered to (32 per cent), suggesting that finding the most workable solutions to lighting issues is more challenging. Changing footwear had over 50 per cent adherence, and changing habitual behaviour was still excellent at over 55 per cent (including things such as accessing steps in a safer manner, or changing the way in which the person reached for objects from higher shelves).

---

26 Lally & Gardner, 2013.
27 Clemson, Cumming, et al., 2004.
28 Cumming, Thomas, et al., 1999.
29 Cumming, Thomas, et al., 1999.

SAFETY GUIDELINES WHEN USING A LADDER

You don't have to fall far off a ladder to be seriously injured: 1–2 metres can be enough. Fractured limbs, spinal cord damage, severe brain injury or even death can result. The numbers of deaths and serious injuries among older Australians, mainly men, after falling from ladders is increasing.[30] Falls most commonly occur while doing home maintenance, followed by gardening, with overreaching, ladder placement and ladder instability implicated in many falls. Men at or near retirement age are in the highest risk category for this type of accident. Stay alert when using a ladder and stay safe.

Check the ladder before use:

- Check the ladder is in good condition, without signs of warping, rust, corrosion or missing rivets.
- Check that non-slip safety feet are fitted and are in good condition.
- Check that the ladder's height is right for the job – if using an extension ladder to access a roof or work area, the top of the ladder should extend at least one metre over the top of the surface on which it is resting.

Set-up:

- Place the ladder on dry, firm, level ground – if the soil is too soft, place a hard board under the ladder's feet to stop it sinking.
- Engage all locks and braces – stepladders should be fully opened.
- Keep the ladder clear of powerlines and exposed electrical wiring.
- The foot of an extension ladder should be placed at a distance from the wall equal to one-quarter of the length of the ladder.

Climb safely:

- Wear good-fitting, enclosed, slip-resistant footwear – not sandals or thongs.
- Have someone hold the ladder at the base while you are using it.

---

30 Vallmuur, Eley, & Watson, 2016.

- Hold the ladder with both hands as you climb, and carry tools in a tool belt.
- Stay in the centre of the ladder as you climb.
- Only climb to the second rung from the top of a stepladder, or the third rung from the top of an extension ladder.
- Secure the top of an extension ladder into position before starting work.

Work safely:

- Work within arm's reach of the ladder – if you cannot easily reach, climb down and re-position the ladder.
- Always hold the ladder with at least one hand.
- Be careful when pulling items from shelves, gutters or roofs, as this may cause you to lose your balance.
- When you are finished, store the ladder in a dry place to prevent warping and corrosion.

Caution:

- Don't take a risk by taking short cuts.
- Never lean a ladder on an unstable or slippery surface.
- Do not walk the ladder while still on it. Climb down and re-position the ladder closer to the work.
- Do not push or pull against other objects when up the ladder, unless the ladder is properly secured – these forces can destabilise the ladder.
- Do not use a ladder if you are working in wind or rain.
- Do not use a ladder if you are affected by medication or if you have a medical condition that can cause you to lose your balance.
- Never have more than one person on the ladder at a time.

REFLECTIONS OF PAULA, ONE OF OUR NEW CO-FACILITATORS FOR THE STEPPING ON PROGRAM

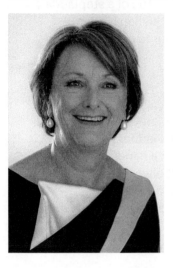

When you have young children and you have a problem, you think you are the only one with that problem, and you go to mothers/fathers group and find there are many more people with that problem – you feel better for that.

In the same way, on the first day of a Stepping On program you are introduced to other group members. Quickly you find out their story, their experiences with falls and their resulting lack of confidence. Straight away you know you are not alone – you feel better for that.

When the Stepping On group leader tells you that you have fallen because you have weak muscles, and that muscles start to deteriorate at a certain age, then tells you that you can turn that situation around, do your exercises and improve – you feel better for that.

When the Stepping On group leader tells you that your balance deteriorates from an even younger age, and you can turn that around by doing your exercises – you feel better for that.

When you come out of your home and possible loneliness and isolation, and possibly little routine, to meet some nice people from your area on a regular basis for 7 weeks, possibly starting new social connections – you feel better for that.

So before you do any regular exercise tasks at all, your confidence and feeling of wellbeing have improved already.

You have already achieved so much from the program, because you feel better, feel more confident and more able to take control of your future and connect with your community.

THE APPLE GAME QUIZ

Use this quiz to generate discussion and problem-solving. We gave apples, which symbolise health and, in Chinese communities, represent safety and health. There can be more than one right answer, depending on the context for the person. The real aim is to problem-solve and discuss the various solutions.

'Choose the answer that will best help prevent a fall for you. You can choose more than one answer. Think about what you do, what you could do, what the barriers might be, and what would make it easier to follow through and do it.'

To answer my phone, I:

(a) go as fast as I can in case they hang up
(b) carefully check that the route to the phone is free of clutter
(c) move slowly and carefully. I leave a window open to hear the phone when I'm outside
(d) don't worry if I don't make it
(e) ask for a cordless phone for my birthday.

I place my heater in winter:

(a) in front of my easy chair to keep me warm
(b) right out of the way of where I walk
(c) near the wall, but with the cord across the floor.

In the bedroom, I:

(a) let the bedclothes trail over the edge of the bed
(b) check the floor space and the route where I walk for clutter
(c) leave the cord from the television across the floor
(d) leave my shoes in front of the window that I open most frequently.

To make steps safer, I:

(a) go down as quickly as possible
(b) get a rail installed
(c) improve the lighting at the top and bottom of the stairs
(d) don't leave clutter on the steps.

So that I don't fall over a cord across the floor, I:

    (a) do not use extension cords
    (b) put tape over the extension cord
    (c) rearrange the furniture so the cord is not across the floor
    (d) use extra cords so they go further
    (e) tape or clip the cord to the walls so that it is not on the floor
    (f) get plug sockets installed where I need them.

To make the outside pathways safer, I:

    (a) get the bushes cut back to clear the path
    (b) use an 'anti-moss' product from the hardware store
    (c) don't go out alone
    (d) install a handrail
    (e) get someone to repair the uneven path.

When I get up at night, I:

    (a) never switch on a night-light
    (b) have a 'touch' lamp beside the bed
    (c) leave a torch beside the bed
    (d) already have a 'photosensitive' light plugged in somewhere along the route to the toilet.

To change a light bulb, I:

    (a) use a stepladder with a firm base and a safety rail to hold onto
    (b) use the kitchen stool to climb on
    (c) put the dining chair on the table and climb up
    (d) ask someone else to do it.

To make sure the pets are not hazardous, I:

    (a) feed the pets by the back door just where I walk out
    (b) get rid of the pet because I might trip over it
    (c) shut them up in the back room at times when I'm really busy
    (d) make sure that my dog is not in the way of the steps when I go out the back door.

My favourite chair:

(a) has lots of soft and slippery cushions to make it cosy
(b) has a footstool in front of the chair to put my feet on
(c) has a mat in front of the chair to stop the carpet wearing
(d) is high enough and has good armrests for standing up easily
(e) is a challenging height for me and reminds me to do my sit-to-stand exercises.

To stop me tripping or slipping on a mat, I:

(a) remove all floor mats
(b) tack or tape down all mats
(c) use purple mats as they are less slippery
(d) use a slip-resistant underlay beneath slippery mats.

To make the kitchen floor safer, I:

(a) remove all rugs
(b) wipe up spills right away
(c) buy a heavy slip-resistant mat
(d) walk carefully in the kitchen.

To make it safer on dim days and at night, I:

(a) increase the wattage of the bulbs I buy
(b) paint the walls a contrasting colour so I can see the furniture
(c) wear dark sunglasses
(d) move furniture out of walkways.

To make it safer when moving about, I:

(a) pause when going from a dim room to a well-lit area
(b) paint the edge of steps with a contrasting strip
(c) always wear my bifocals when walking around the house
(d) get infrared glasses for night-time walks.

To move safely from the kitchen to my lounge chair, I:

(a) have lots of furniture and things to hold onto
(b) get rid of my old large dining table as it is too big and the chairs are in the way
(c) leave the low coffee table with splayed legs in the middle of the room.

Reaching to high shelves, I:

    (a) have my most-used items in easy reach
    (b) use my cane to pull down things I can't reach
    (c) have higher shelves painted a darker colour
    (d) put the things I often have to reach up for onto a lower shelf.

To make my bath safer, I:

    (a) use a rubber bath mat inside the bath
    (b) install grab bars
    (c) get rid of my bathtub and put in a shower
    (d) paint my bath yellow because this is a safe colour.

To make my bathroom floor safer, I:

    (a) remove all the mats
    (b) replace the mats frequently when worn
    (c) paint the floor with a non-slip substance so it is less
        slippery when wet
    (d) always wear stockings or socks in the bathroom
    (e) use talcum powder.

When I don't need my walking stick, I:

    (a) put it down against the nearest wall or table
    (b) always check it is safely placed so that I won't trip over it
    (c) use a 'walking stick holder' when I go out.

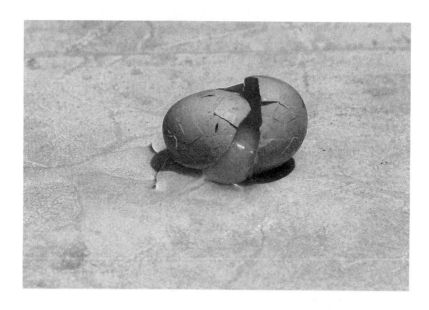

HOME FALLS HAZARDS SLIDES

The 'Home Falls Hazards' slides are available for download from the Sydney University Press website (sydneyuniversitypress.com.au/stepping-on-2019). The following notes can be used to discuss the 'Home Falls Hazards' slides.

1. 'Home falls hazards'
2. Where do you think falls occur the most?
3. In the living area?
4. What about where injurious falls occur?
5. Falls with injuries also occur in living areas and in wet areas like bathrooms.
6. Falls occur indoors and outdoors.
7. What time of day do falls occur?
8. Late morning and late afternoon – when most busy and before a meal.
9. List of the most common hazards in fall studies.
10. List of the most common hazards in fall studies.
11. Solutions: change things around the home or change the way you do things.
12. Look at the following pictures. What is the hazard? What could be your solution?
13. Slippery floors and wet areas are at the top of our hazard list. What would be some of the potentially slippery areas, or at what times might there be some slippery hazards in your home? Wipe up spills straight away.
14. Egg – wipe up with detergent and hot water.
15. A spill on the floor. Butter, oils and water are most dangerous. What to do? Wipe up right away and use detergent if oil or lubricant involved.

    'My husband came in from the garden and fell in the kitchen as he turned. He is a large man and came down heavily on his side. I had dropped a knife with butter and quickly wiped the excess off with a paper cloth, but had failed to do a good enough job because I did not take the time to use a detergent. Now I always make sure I get rid of grease or oil properly.'

16. Clutter in the living room. Avoid footrests.
17. The dragging bedspread cover and the shoes in the walkway. The shoes on the bedroom floor are a good example of a habit that is hard to break. One of our ladies fell over a shoe and then she remembered this slide. She has worked at changing that habit now.

18. Darkness in doorways. Point out that this is at the end of a stairwell. There is dark brown carpet on the hall floor, a stairwell coming down from the left and another hall beyond it. The dimness and dark floor make it impossible to see the step coming the other way. Clutter at doorways. Telephone in a difficult position and nowhere to sit.

19. Poor visibility in stairwell and slippery wooden steps. Put in lighting or use the lights that are there. Have a two-way light switch installed. Install a skylight if possible. Paint walls a lighter colour. Put indoor non-slip treads on steps in a contrasting colour. All of these things were actually done over a period of time to improve this stairwell.

20. Standing on a chair. Anyone admit to doing this? What about changing a light bulb? What are the alternatives? Show a set of steps and ask people to pick out safety features. Discuss storage of ladder (it is lightweight and foldable, but if not stored in a handy position we won't use it).

21. Mossy, slippery steps. Hose at gate. No rail at steps.

22. Going to the bathroom at night. A photosensitive light can be left on all the time. It responds to darkness and only comes on at night to softly light up a pathway. You don't have to rely on your memory to turn it on each night. It's not a brilliant light to wake you, and it's cheap and can be bought at the supermarket, along with replacement bulbs.

23. Cord across the floor and sitting at a table in the doorway. Need to relocate the light and also the table. Perhaps it could be moved flush with the wall now, as only the couple lives at home.

24. Steps and stairs. Woman holding dog walking down steps without holding handrail. Our actions can put us at risk.

25. This is more dangerous due to the light and shadows.

26. Long dressing-gown. Take particular care coming down steps in long and loose clothing. (Use a real dressing-gown as a cue.)

27. Green hose on green grass.

28. Reaching and leaning forward or up too high.

29. Hallway clutter in walkways; obstacles to answering the door; loose mat on a slippery floor.

30. Lighting; pot plants in walkways; pot plants dropping leaves and flowers; obstacles in the walkways so have to move to other side to get down; no handrail.

31. Overreaching on ladder; too high; no one else at home; ladder not on secure footing; always done it; difficult to accept to ask someone else.

32. Now let's revise: What is the hazard? It can be an object or a behaviour. How to fix it? What are the barriers to getting it done? How to keep it going? Refer to homework for next week.

Table: Home fall hazard screening checklist*

QUESTION	YES	NO	COMMENTS
Are the bathroom or kitchen floors slippery when wet or dry?			
Are there any obstacles in walkways indoors, on stairs, steps, or on outside pathways?			
Is the lighting dim or shadowy in living areas, walkways, or stairs?			
Do steps lack colour contrast, have worn coverings, or lack a handrail?			
Are floor mats slippery, loose or have curled edges?			
Are floor coverings worn or loose?			
Are you unsafe when reaching or climbing? Do you use unstable furniture when climbing?			
Do you have a sturdy stepladder?			
Does your footwear fit well and have good fastenings, non-slip soles and a low, wide heel?			
Are your outdoor pathways uneven, broken, loose or mossy?			
Are there cords on the floor?			
Are there spills on the floor? Do you clean up spills straight away?			

SESSION 03

TOPIC

* Home Fall Hazards Screening Checklist (modified from the Westmead Home Safety Assessment, Clemson, 1997). Source: Hill, K., Clemson, L., & Vrantsidis, F. (2006). Preventing falls – a key to maintaining independence. In H. Mackey & S. Nancarrow (Eds.), *Enabling independence – a guide for rehabilitation workers* (pp. 182–202). London: Blackwell.

Alternative checklist 'Staying active and on your feet' is available at www.activeandhealthy.nsw.gov.au/preventing-falls/staying-active -and-on-your-feet

RECOMMENDED READING

Vance, E., Delbaere, K., & Lord, S. (2015). Home safety interventions to prevent falls: a mini review. *Falls Links, NSW Fall Prevention Network*, *10*(4), 2–6.

Home and Community Safety online training modules are available at https://fallspreventiononlineworkshops.com.au/courses/home-and -community-safety

The Westmead Home Safety Assessment (2016) is available under 'Resources tab: Home & Community Safety' at https://fallspreventiononlineworkshops. com.au/tool

Session 4
—
Community safety and footwear

OBJECTIVES

The main objectives of this session are:

1. to raise awareness of the type and range of fall hazards when moving about the local community
2. to increase observation of various fall hazards
3. to generate strategies that will increase personal safety and reduce the risk of falls when moving about the local community
4. to be able to identify the features of a safe shoe
5. to accomplish an audit of shoes at home
6. to identify clothing hazards that can cause a fall.

RESOURCES FOR SESSION 4

Session materials: Session 4 agenda; name tags; attendance sheet; display board and display items; flip chart, butcher's paper or whiteboard; marker pen; door signs; pens for participants to use.

Handouts and flyers: 'Shoe audit'; 'Safe shoe award'; 'Moving about safely: goal-setting checklist'; 'Moving about safely: outdoor walking'; 'Moving about safely: winter mobility tips'; community mobility brochures – as provided by the guest speaker.

Catering: snacks and beverages for break.

Other resources: leg weights; selection of presenters' shoes to demonstrate a shoe audit; collection of 'wacky' shoes and slippers for participants to rate.

PREPARING COMMUNITY SAFETY EXPERT

Photocopy of 4.4 'Community mobility'.

Outline of Session 4: Community safety and footwear

4.1 WELCOME AND OUTLINE 4 MIN	Introductions and brief outline of today's session. Ask the group for three messages they remember from last week. Check homework and collect exercise goals.
4.2 EXERCISE REVIEW AND PRACTICE 10 MIN	Review how to do selected exercises, asking for specific requests. Check participants are fitting the exercises into their daily routines. Advance exercises as able.
4.3 HOME FALLS HAZARDS HOMEWORK 7 MIN	Review the home falls hazards homework. Ask each person to respond.
4.4 COMMUNITY MOBILITY AND SAFETY 40 MIN	Discussion led by guest speaker. Group facilitator recaps major points arising in session.
4.5 FOOTWEAR AND FALLS 35 MIN	Demonstration of hazardous and safe footwear features. The 'Shoe audit' and 'Safe shoe award'.
4.6 HOMEWORK 3 MIN	To determine a goal from the community mobility talk. Ask participants to choose something they could apply at home and tell the group about at next week's session. Suggest selecting light-coloured clothing when going out. Being aware when on a pedestrian crossing. Do a shoe audit at home. If buying a new pair of shoes, try to apply the safety features to the choice.

4.1 WELCOME AND OUTLINE (4 MIN)

Welcome participants and briefly outline the session, letting the group know who the speaker will be.

At the beginning of each week, ask 'What three things do you remember from last week?'

Ask to see the weekly exercise records and check the homework.

4.2 EXERCISE REVIEW AND PRACTICE (10 MIN)

- 'How did the exercises go this week?'
- 'Did you remember how they were done?'
- 'Were they easy to fit into your schedule, or were there any barriers?'
- Review how they are fitting the exercises into their daily routines.
- 'How many times a week are you doing the exercises?'
- 'Has anyone advanced their exercises during the week?'
- Review the exercises, asking for specific requests and questions.

Ask them: 'Which exercises would you like us to go over today?'

Practise some of the exercises. Concentrate on those that people have questions about or find difficult.

Ask the group if someone would like to demonstrate an advanced exercise they did. Advance the exercises and weights as necessary for each exercise the group practises.

It is important to do only a few exercises and review them thoroughly, going over the purpose of the exercise.

4.3 HOME FALLS HAZARDS HOMEWORK (7 MIN)

Review the home falls hazards homework by asking each person to respond: what did they notice, what could be changed, or what has been changed? They may have noticed a loose tile or that the hedge needed trimming. Ask them if they looked at their home falls hazard checklist and what they changed. Did they think of registering for MyAgedCare community services?

Example: Bill was a bachelor. He said his home was just fine, but out in the backyard, where he spends most of his time, he had realised his shed was quite hazardous and needed a lot of reorganisation. He had worked out a plan to do this.

4.4 COMMUNITY MOBILITY AND SAFETY (40 MIN)

(Our guest speaker will complete this section. At the end of the session, hand out 'Moving about safely: goal-setting checklist', and 'Moving about safely: outdoor walking')

For countries and climates that experience snow or ice, also refer to the topic: 'Moving about safely: winter mobility tips' and the associated handout.

Invite a speaker to lead a discussion on community and pedestrian safety. The speaker should be up to date with the current road rules and pedestrian issues. The aim is to find someone with some expertise, familiarity, or interest in this area, so that they can demonstrate the major points in a variety of ways with local examples. These would include the various situations, risks and safety alternatives when getting about the community. Suggestions for speakers are local council road safety officers, or volunteers recommended by state road transport associations. Sometimes speakers can be sourced from community transport services.

Encourage your guest to use a range of ways of illustrating the major points. These can include stories of their experiences, photographs, pictures, facts and figures, and gadgets (e.g. flashlights).

Example: Charles was a volunteer with the Transportation Department. He regularly gave presentations on both pedestrian and driver safety, but we asked him to tailor his discussion for our group to pedestrian safety only. He had points and diagrams on heavy paper made up into a flip chart. He set this up on a chair or table and could flip over to the relevant page. He drew on many stories and examples from real-life situations. We arranged for the purchase of smaller items such as torches and reflective tape.

Note: The speaker or participants may talk about local trouble spots, depending on the living area of the group. However, the focus needs to be directed back to what the individual can do to be safe and not on what the local government should be doing.

People often tell us in the next session about the things they have tried out and the changes they are introducing to their lives.

The risks:

- As we grow older we may not see all the hazards. We need to be more observant.
- Our usual pace may be rushed.
- On the other hand, our pace may be slower than it used to be, or slowed for a medical reason, such as the medication we are taking.
- It may take longer to cross the road.
- It may be more difficult to see in low light conditions.
- We may not hear traffic, or traffic noise may be confusing.
- Crossing the road on a diagonal takes longer and we are less likely to be seen.
- Crossing the road in front of parked cars makes us less visible to drivers.
- Uneven pavements, pavers and footpaths are a common problem.
- Slippery areas are a concern – slippery surfaces, wet areas, and particularly supermarket floors.
- Kerbs, gutters and ramps may be becoming difficult to negotiate.
- Take extra care at uncontrolled intersections, by which we mean intersections with no traffic lights, road markings or signs to indicate who has right of way. The traffic may give confusing signals, and no two drivers seem to indicate the same way.
- We may have trouble gauging the speed of cars.

The strategies, and some ways of emphasising and illustrating the strategies:

- Don't ever be in a hurry. Plan so that it is not necessary to rush.
- When participants express concern about being knocked or jostled in crowds, encourage:
  - mobility practice
  - strengthening the legs and improving balance through exercise
  - using a shopping trolley around the shopping centre
  - having their vision checked.

Crossing streets:

- Never assume the driver has seen you when you're about to cross the road. Make eye contact with the driver. It's also a good idea to acknowledge you have seen them stop. Even if you can't see them clearly, look towards the driver. This is a definite communication that you want to cross and that they should stop or remain stationary.

- Cross away from where there are parked cars and other visual obstructions to motorists. Move to where you can be seen. Walk that extra bit.
- Cross with other people if possible.
- Walk to the traffic lights. The exercise is good. A flashing red pedestrian light indicates that people should not leave the kerb, but if you have already begun crossing the road and it is safe to do so, you can continue crossing. It is not meant to tell you to rush. People often tell us they are very nervous crossing because they feel the light is flashing at them – they have to remind themselves that it is not meant for them, but for people who haven't yet started to cross.
- When going out on dark or cloudy days, at dusk or at night – or to ensure that you are clearly seen at *any* time:
  - **Wear light-coloured clothing and carry a yellow or light-coloured umbrella.** We tend to wear dark or basic colours that make it more difficult for drivers to see us. To illustrate this: use a picture, or look outside and spot the older person in light-coloured clothing, or look around the room and see who would pass the *being seen* test.
  - **Carry a torch at dusk and at night.** Have a selection on display (see 'The display' in 'Part 3: Resources').
  - **Put reflective tape around your bag, walking stick or arm.** This can be purchased from bicycle shops.
- Windy days are a concern. Take extra care or avoid going out on windy days – stand with your legs apart to give a wider 'base of support'.
- If you need them, wear your glasses and hearing aid when outdoors.
- Carry a walking stick and people will look out for you.
- Look around and choose the path with the least number of hazards. (Use the outside of the venue to illustrate this. Which way is the best way to go? What are your alternatives? The quickest route is not always the safest.)
- Scan a few metres ahead when you walk. Don't look straight down or far away. Scanning ahead gives you time to adjust your step and to avoid a trip or slip hazard. Refer to the therapist's presentation.
- Walk down kerb ramps with a wider leg base for support.
- When there are gutters or kerbs to negotiate, try to pick a spot where there is a pole to hold for support.

- Hold your bag safely over your shoulder and walk close to walls if you are concerned about bag-snatching.

4.5　FOOTWEAR AND FALLS (35 MIN)

(Hand out the 'Shoe audit' and the 'What is a safe, comfortable shoe?' handouts.)

Demonstration of hazardous and safe footwear features

We first use a selection of our own shoes to demonstrate the 'Shoe audit' and the hazardous and safe features, and then we provide a collection of 'wacky' and other assorted shoes and slippers for participants to audit. Participants are then more willing to talk about the shoes they are wearing, even if they are unsafe. The purpose is to encourage them to identify and learn the features of a safe shoe and then to apply this knowledge by doing a shoe audit. We clean and sterilise (in the sun) all second-hand shoes and let people know that we have done so. Be sure to explain that shoes are a personal choice and that you understand this. However, there are lots of options for safer shoes. It's important to recognise when your shoes or slippers are unsafe.

The presenter displays a selection of footwear that they currently wear (or have replaced) and asks the group to say what is unsafe and what is good about each example. We used a slipper, an everyday shoe, a dress shoe and some joggers.

We refer to the 'four-point audit': support, sole, heel and fit (written on the whiteboard or flip chart) throughout the discussion. We are looking for hazardous features, and safety features and solutions (see the 'What is a safe, comfortable shoe' handouts). For each shoe, ask the group:

- What's safe about this shoe?
- What's not so good about this one?
- What could I do about it?

Let the participants come up with the features and respond positively. Prompt them by adding some useful ideas as you go along. Give an idea or solution and wait for a reaction. Participants will support it or not and will add solutions of their own.

Molly laughed at our 'wacky' stiletto shoe. She joked about the days when she and her best friend would get all dressed up on Friday nights. 'We would put on our stilettos,' she said. 'We called them "Man Catchers", and we'd race up to the city in them.'

This exercise requires the presenter to be honest.

Display your worn slippers that need to be replaced because they offer so little support that they make you shuffle as you walk.

Or explain how you bought these shoes because the sole had a good grip when you first bought them (having a textured and broken pattern), but did not notice till you did the audit how worn they have become. This gives no protection from a slip. Explain what you intend to do.

'The joggers have good, safe ties, a firm arch support, and are a good fit. But they have thick soles – they are made for running or jumping. Do you run or jump? I don't either! The thick soles are easier to trip on, especially on stairs. So, a better choice is a walking shoe that has a firm but thinner sole to give better feedback from what you are standing on.'

'These good shoes look fantastic, but the heels are too high and unstable, and there is no support. I have to begin to accept that I need something safer for those nights out.'

'These shoes were expensive but have a smooth leather sole. What can I do to make them safer before I wear them?'

Offer your comments as the group comes up with answers, or to prompt other ideas.

Refer to the 'What is a safe, comfortable shoe' handout (or poster) and recap the safety features.

Footwear audit

The participants are now each given a shoe or slipper from the 'assorted and wacky collection', a 'Shoe audit' handout and a pen. This segment is usually fun, and it seems to get the main messages across. We used fluffy slippers, stiletto heels, worn-down heels, loafers, slip-ons, worn men's shoes – any example that accentuates a hazardous feature.

'Tick the "Shoe audit" only if the shoe meets the safety standard for stability, fit, sole and heel. Only tick it if it is safe. Add up how many ticks each shoe gets.'

Make sure everyone knows what has to be done next. Repeat the instructions individually if need be and help people get started.

When the task is completed ask each person the results of their audit. Then ask the group to suggest who gave the best answer. That person receives the 'Safe shoe award'.

See also:

- footwear in 'Footwear, feet and falls' topic
- handouts: 'What is a safe, comfortable shoe?'; 'Shoe audit'; 'Moving about safely: winter mobility tips' and 'Yaktrax walker ice and snow grips'.

4.6 HOMEWORK (3 MIN)

End with the homework suggestions:

- Apply something participants learned from the community mobility talk that they want to try on their own and tell the group about at next week's session. Suggest selecting light-coloured clothing when going out.
- Suggest participants do a shoe audit at home on their own shoes using the four-point audit. Hand out an extra sheet to take home and bring back to the next session. If buying a new pair of shoes, try to apply the safety features, and share how this went with the group next time.

Indicate the topics for the following week:

- vision and falls
- vitamin D and calcium.

Footwear, feet and falls

Unsafe footwear and the increased chance of foot problems associated with ageing can both contribute to falls.

Age-related changes to our feet include thinner, dryer skin that is less resilient to friction and more likely to get corns and calluses, soft tissue (such as in our heels) that is less shock absorbent, decreased muscle mass with reduced strength (such as in our toes, which we need for gripping as we move forward), reduced range of motion in our ankles, and (finally!) increasing proneness to dropped arches and 'flat feet', which is one reason why gait can be slower and steps smaller. Foot problems impair balance, placing people at higher risk of falls.[1] Further, independent risk factors for falls[2] include foot pain, hallux valgus ('bunions'), lesser toe deformity (hammer-toe and claw-toe), weak toe flexors, and a reduced range of motion in the ankle.

But the good news is that the Foothold trial[3] is the first study to have shown a significant reduction in falls through a 'footwear and feet' intervention, demonstrating a 36 per cent reduction in the rate of falls. The intervention impressively improved ankle strength, range of motion, and postural sway (balance) and had a positive trend towards reducing pain. The intervention was comprised of three key components: advice on footwear, foot orthoses, and a home-based program of foot and ankle exercises, along with a booklet on general fall prevention.

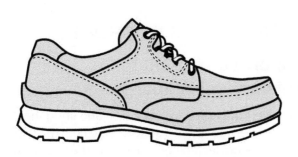

We refer you to a recorded presentation by Professor Hylton Menz of La Trobe University for more in-depth background to this section:
www.foothold.org.au

---

1   Menz, Morris, & Lord, 2005.
2   Menz, Morris, & Lord, 2006; Mickle, Munro, et al., 2009; Mickle, Munro, et al., 2010.
3   Spink, Menz, et al., 2011.

FOOTWEAR

We teach people how to do an 'audit' of their shoes: to know the features of a safe shoe and also what features make shoes unsafe. We encourage them to keep in mind these features when buying new shoes. Most people's shoes are well used and worn. What was once a safe shoe may no longer give support, and the heel and sole will probably be worn and slippery. Yet this is a risk that can go unnoticed. Information on home repair kits and paint-on rubber soling solutions (see 'Part 3: Resources' – 'the display') are alternatives to expensive repairs. Try them out on your own shoes so that you can speak from experience.

Shoes are personal. People buy them for both comfort and fashion, so talk about comfort, fashion and safety. Do you turn the shoe over and inspect the sole when buying shoes? Is that on your list of what to look for? Try to think of the purpose for which you are buying the shoe (e.g. walking) so that you don't lose sight of the need for practicality. Keep fashion buying under control! When buying for fashion, try a good brand that is well made, with a supportive, firm arch support. Price, however, is not necessarily a good indicator of safety features. For example, some expensive shoes have slippery leather soles. What could you do to make a leather sole safer? Scoring with a file or using the non-slip rubber soling solution are two options.

We need to consider indoor shoes, outdoor shoes and slippers. Many falls at home have occurred when people were wearing slippers,[4] and some older people wear slippers at home for the majority of the day. Less attention is generally paid to slippers or to the replacement of worn slippers than to shoes, yet worn slippers will contribute to shuffling and do not encourage heel-and-toe walking.

Shoes and slippers need to be stable and supportive, offer a good fit, and have a sole and heel that grip.

THE SAFETY FEATURES OF SHOES

A supportive shoe that fits well provides stability

A supportive shoe covers most of the foot and has a firm and snug 'heel counter', a reinforcement of the heel cup. Such a shoe should hold the foot well back into the shoe and have secure fastenings. Fastening the shoe with laces or Velcro ensures the shoe 'holds' onto the foot when walking. Slip-ons are very unsafe and contribute to poor gait, particularly if the toes need

---

4   Finlay, 1986.

to grip tightly to hold the shoe on. A study of people admitted to hospital following hip fracture showed that those who tripped were three times more likely to have been wearing shoes without fixation.[5] A supportive shoe with a firm arch offers stability. A midsole that is flexible under the ball of the foot and not too thick will offer comfort and will allow proprioceptive sensory feedback, which also contributes to stability. Sensory and motor feedback provide information on where the foot is and what surface it is on. This is particularly important on stairs and other changes in levels. Many joggers and sneakers are comfortable, but have a thick undersole that does not offer the same degree of safety. These shoes are made for shock attenuation so that they are suitable for running, but for everyday walking, a walking shoe that is lightweight, thinner-soled and flexible is the best choice. This can be a trade-off for some people, who find the thicker softer midsole comfortable, but the stiffer midsole does impair balance and even 'stopping' ability.[6] There are exceptions when a thicker sole is indicated, e.g. thicker, softer midsoles are important for people with diabetic neuropathy.

A firm and relatively high heel collar is advised for stability because it has been shown to improve mechanical stability and also has a tactile proprioceptive effect where it grasps around the ankle.[7]

When buying shoes, have your feet measured properly so that the shoe fits well. It needs to have a roomy toe box to prevent foot deformity and to give comfort. We recommend elastic shoelaces and a long-handled shoehorn to enable a person to don their own supportive shoes.

A sole that grips and a heel that is stable and grips

Most slips occur at heel strike, so the rear of the heel is particularly important. The heel needs to be textured for traction, with a pattern and depth that will penetrate any spills or lubricant on the floor and will grip less-resistant surfaces. A bevelled heel, in which the rear section is cut away, offers a good flat surface for gripping at heel strike. This is a good, safe feature that is becoming easier to find, though less so for women's shoes. Broader heels and a bevelled heel were proven important in laboratory studies testing the coefficient of friction of men's shoes and ladies' court shoes on various surfaces.[8] They found that some features were important in dry conditions, but no features improved safety on wet surfaces.

---

5   Sherrington & Menz, 2003.
6   Menant, Steele, et al., 2008.
7   Menant, Steele, et al., 2009a; Menant, Steele, et al., 2009b.
8   Menz, Lord, & McIntosh, 2001.

A low, broad heel is essential for stability[9] and is negatively associated with falling.[10] However, women used to wearing high heels should not suddenly go into flat shoes as their tendons will be constricted. Instead, they will need to adapt gradually to a lower heel. There are other exceptions – for example people with a reduced range of ankle movement may have difficulty in a flat shoe. Non-slip socks have been shown to be a better alternative to bare feet indoors.[11] Some socks have rubber grip 'dots' to prevent slipping. It has been suggested that they would be particularly good for older people with a slower gait.

Be wary of smooth-soled shoes.

Foot orthoses to improve comfort and minimise pressure spots

Foot orthoses were an important component of the Foothold trial, which recruited people who had a history of foot pain. In that trial, the participants were offered 'off-the-shelf' orthoses (which are easily accessible, e.g. Formthotics™) to people who were not already wearing customised or prefabricated orthoses. They were heat-moulded to the shape of the person's foot. If there were calluses or other plantar lesions, then padding (Poron®) was placed underneath the insole in the area needing padding. The investigators reported[12] that they believed the foot orthoses had a direct effect on balance (because they improved foot stability and enhanced sensory feedback) and an indirect effect (by reducing pressure and reducing foot pain). Balance issues and foot pain have both been implicated in falls.

There are a range of off-the-shelf orthotics available via the internet or local pharmacists. Podiatrists, occupational therapists or physiotherapists would also be able to provide advice for those with severe foot deformity.

PODIATRY

Falls prevention guidelines recommend referral to a podiatrist; however, there is a great deal of variability in podiatry treatments offered. Foot care, callus reduction and foot-care education are indicated as helpful. These issues could be managed by regular visits to (or home visits by) the podiatrist for foot care (e.g. for bunions, hammer toes, calluses and painful feet), or by referral to an orthotist if required. The www.foothold. org.au website is highly recommended for podiatrists and other health

---

9   Menant, Steele, et al., 2009a.
10   Tencer, Koepsell, et al., 2004.
11   Hatton, Sturnieks, et al., 2013.
12   Spink, Menz, et al., 2011.

professionals who wish to be updated on evidence-based foot and footwear falls prevention interventions.

FOOT AND ANKLE EXERCISES TO PREVENT FALLS

If people have weak ankles or foot pain, refer them to the evidence-based FootHold website. The FootHold exercises were design to improve ankle and foot flexibility and strength (see www.foothold.org.au). The website has a video showing the exercises. The trial participants were asked to perform the exercises three times a week. Participants self-managed upgrading their exercises by increasing repetitions and/or resistance. They did this at their own pace. The exercises contributed to the positive trial outcomes.

Provide information on the FootHold website for those interested.

RECOMMENDED READING

Lord, S. R., Sherrington, C., & Menz, H. B. (2007). Chapter 10. The role of footwear in falls prevention. In *Falls in older people: risk factors and strategies for prevention*. Cambridge, UK: Cambridge University Press.

WALKERS FOR WALKING IN ICE AND SNOW CONDITIONS

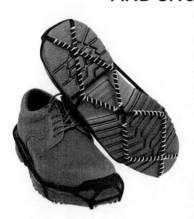

The Yaktrax Walk snow and ice grips are a simple walking device that improves stability and reduces falls in hazardous winter conditions. They stretch to fit over your regular shoes, are lightweight and inexpensive, and are available online or at sporting goods stores in countries with cold climates. They have a coil design that increases traction when walking over packed snow or ice, keeping you from slipping. You can keep them in your purse, pocket or glove compartment because they only weigh 160 g (5.6 ounces) and have no sharp edges. Yaktrax won't damage most floors, but you shouldn't wear them indoors!

No product can guarantee that you won't fall, but a study published by the American Geriatrics Society in June 2005 confirmed that the Yaktrax Walker can reduce outdoor winter falls and help to keep older adults safer on ice and snow.

Session 5
—
Vision, transportation safety, vitamin D & calcium

OBJECTIVES

The main objectives of this session are:

1. to understand how vision can influence the ability to get around safely
2. to plan regular vision checks
3. to explore functional adaptations that will help reduce falls hazards due to poor vision
4. to understand defensive walking and how to scan ahead
5. to list safety strategies for safe bus and train travel
6. to understand the importance of calcium and vitamin D as protection against falls and fall injuries
7. to become aware of the importance of weekly exposure to sunlight.

RESOURCES FOR SESSION 5

Session materials: Session 5 agenda; name tags; attendance sheet; display board and display items; flip chart, butcher's paper or whiteboard; marker pen; door signs.

Handouts and flyers: 'Vision and falling'; 'Sun time checklist'; 'Vitamin D'; 'Calcium checklist for one day'; 'Bus travel safety' and 'Train travel safety' handouts, depending on local needs of participants.

Catering: snacks and beverages for break.

Other resources: leg weights; walking stick, sunglasses and other mobility vision aids as requested by vision expert; lighting samples and reflective tape; bowl, detergent and dirty spectacles; information on local low-vision support groups/clinics/agencies.

PREPARING VISION EXPERT

Copy section 5.3, 'Vision and falls', and the topic section titled 'Vision and falls'.

Outline of Session 5: Vision, vitamin D, calcium and travel safety

5.1 WELCOME AND OUTLINE 4 MIN	Welcome participants. Ask the group for three messages they remember from last week. Discuss the homework and check weekly exercise records. Introduce the day's program and the guest speaker.
5.2 REVIEW OF HOMEWORK AND EXERCISES 15 MIN	Review personal goals and achievements with pedestrian safety since the previous week. 'Did anyone try a shoe audit or shop for shoes? How did that go?' Review exercises and practise difficult ones. Review how participants are fitting the exercises into their daily lives. Ask how the weights are going and upgrade if needed.
5.3 VISION AND FALLS 35 MIN	Guest expert to lead participatory-style presentation. Facilitator to recap important points. Invite further questions during the break and follow up appointments if needed.
BREAK 15 MIN	
5.4 REFLECTIONS OF A FORMER PARTICIPANT 5 MIN	Guest participant from a former group to talk about what he/she gained from the program, and their personal barriers and achievements.
5.5 VITAMIN D, CALCIUM AND SUNLIGHT 20 MIN	Discussion: questions and answers.
5.6 TRAVEL SAFETY 15 MIN	Brainstorm strategies on transportation safety.

5.7 HOMEWORK 4 MIN	'Determine a personal goal based on today's experiences. Apply something you want to try, and tell the group next week how you went.'
	'Plan being in the sun for 10–15 minutes about every second day. Take home the "Sun time checklist", and tick it off during the week.' Remind participants to complete the weekly exercise records.
	Gear up for the following week. Tell everyone about the final therapist visit next week, and the choice they can make between the mobility mastery practice and the video/discussion.

5.1 WELCOME AND OUTLINE (4 MIN)

Always ask the participants for three things they can remember from last week.

Make introductions and give a brief outline of today's session.

Check the weekly exercise records.

5.2 REVIEW OF HOMEWORK AND EXERCISES (15 MIN)

- Review participants' personal goals and achievements regarding pedestrian safety during the preceding week.
- Review the shoe audit homework.

Did anyone try a shoe audit or shop for shoes? How did that go?

- Review the exercises and practise difficult ones. Link these exercises to how they prevent falls and improve function.
- Ask how participants are fitting the exercises into their daily lives.
- Ask how the weights are going and increase if needed.
- Ask if someone would like to demonstrate an advanced exercise they can do.
- Recognise individual achievements. Some people don't like to be told what to do. For example, one participant told us she was doing the exercises voluntarily because 'You didn't

tell me I had to do it for the rest of my life.' It is important that people figure that out for themselves. Positively reinforce her efforts. 'It's fantastic that you're achieving this in your everyday life.' Praise and support is important from the facilitator and often spontaneous from other group members.

- Ask for ideas about why it is important to keep the exercises challenging.

5.3. VISION AND FALLS (35 MIN)

It is ideal if the guest speaker is an expert in conducting orientation and mobility training for people with vision loss. Vision is a neglected area in falls prevention. People are often unaware of declining vision and tend to adapt unconsciously to changing vision. This may not always be a safe way to deal with it. It is important to raise awareness about the implications of vision impairment, to introduce safety strategies, and to encourage participants to plan regular eye check-ups.

The major vision and falls messages from the research are (see Session 5 'Topics' for more detailed background information):

- Don't ignore changes to your vision.
- Have eye tests at least every two years.
- Wear glasses and update them regularly. Take particular care when being mobile outdoors with new lenses, because you need time to adapt to the changes.
- Have timely cataract surgery when needed.
- Get a referral to a low-vision clinic if required.
- There are adaptations for coping with vision loss in negotiating the home, outdoor and community environments.

Invite a guest expert to lead an interactive discussion on vision and falls. This person needs to be an expert on orientation and mobility strategies for vision loss, and able to answer specific questions about individual eye conditions and provide some resources to demonstrate the major points in different ways.

Facilitators provide the speaker with the necessary information about falls prevention so they can be prepared for the link between vision and falls. This is more about coping with low vision, and reference to specific conditions such as macular degeneration needs to be relevant to the group participants. The fact sheet 'Vision and falls' will provide background information.

Suggestions for guest vision experts are a representative of a vision organisation such as the Guide Dogs Association, an optometrist with geriatric experience, or an ophthalmologist interested in the issue of falls prevention. We were assisted by orientation and mobility specialists from the Guide Dogs Association of NSW and by Vision Australia, who were trained in strategies to cope with low vision. The session was specifically crafted around falls and low vision.

Encourage your guest to use a range of ways to illustrate the major points. For example, pictures of views simulating different eye conditions have been particularly useful for our participants. Comparing the vision-impaired view with the unimpaired view can give a clear understanding of the impact that vision has on our ability to avoid trip and slip hazards. Having a range of sunglasses to show different sunglass tints that accommodate for different eye conditions is another useful prompt.

An interactive session on vision and falls

(Presented by the vision expert)

1. Introduction: vision conditions and falls risk. Briefly introduce the types of vision conditions and their falls risk.

Ask people from the group about the vision conditions they have and help them make the link to potential fall situations. Invite questions and answers and use visual illustrations (see comments below) – note that this is not a presentation of all possible conditions. The kinds of conditions may include changes accompanying ageing, such as not clearly seeing edges with contrast sensitivity, which happens with most eyesight problems, being more aware that glare affects one's ability to see things on a pathway, and problems associated with a specific condition (e.g. macular degeneration – only use this example if someone in group can relate to this condition).

Briefly discuss some of the side effects of those conditions mentioned. Be as interactive as possible, encouraging the participants to relate their personal experiences, or use a story from a typical case study.

Visual illustrations (e.g. photographs or everyday practical examples) of different conditions causing impaired vision compared with normal vision are useful in generating awareness.

The aim in this introduction is to raise awareness of how visual loss can exacerbate the difficulties in getting around, such as in getting up and down steps and kerbs when wearing bifocals, or the way conditions like cataracts make it harder to see trip hazards or changes in levels. The introduction leads on to the subsequent sections.

There are some relatively simple and straightforward things that can be done to reduce the risk of falls associated with visual loss: for example, having regular eye checks, walking defensively, using visual aids, or simple functional adaptations like wearing a hat to reduce glare.

2. Regular eye check-ups. When was the last time you had your vision checked? Many people could greatly benefit from a change in glasses. Regular eye check-ups (at least once every two years) with an eye specialist or optometrist are essential. This is highly recommended by researchers in falls prevention. Discuss what financial support is available. Medicare allows bulk-billed check-ups every year for people who are 65 and over. This will help you to keep across your eye health at a time when your eyes are changing rapidly.

> **Vision**
>
> We all get used to living with 'not quite perfect' eyesight – we learn to live with it. So:
>
> 1. Have your eyes checked at least every two years by an eye specialist or optometrist. Many of us would see much better with new glasses.
> 2. Clean your glasses regularly. They get very dirty just by being used. This can be done with soap or detergent in the kitchen sink, or even in the shower. You'll be amazed at the difference! Use the cloths available from optometrist shops or chemists. Don't use tissues before washing your glasses well as that can scratch your glasses lenses.

Regular eye checks can lead to diagnosing more severe conditions. Gerry came back to many of our groups to discuss his experiences. He had had undiagnosed glaucoma for a long time and now has tunnel vision. He emphasised that this would have been avoidable with regular check-ups.

> **When you get new glasses, take care moving around outdoors**
>
> You can be at risk of a fall, so be extra careful until you get used to the new lenses. Take your time, hold onto the rails or other street furniture to steady yourself, and be vigilant about scanning ahead as you 'heel-and-toe' walk and negotiate kerbs and steps.

3. Timely cataract surgery. Cataracts can make it difficult to see when moving about, and research shows a link between cataracts and falls. Falls research recommends surgical intervention for cataracts as soon as possible. Tell participants: 'If you have cataracts and have had a fall, it would be beneficial to see your doctor to initiate an early referral for cataract treatment.'

Some lighting conditions, such as glare, can also make it more difficult to see with cataracts.

Photos demonstrating cataract conditions can highlight how cataracts can make it difficult to see the edges of steps and paths.

4. Safe mobility outside. Demonstrate where possible. Relate the following to prevention:

- Defensive walking – scanning ahead for hazards, 'eyeballing' the motorists when crossing roads, and other strategies. These are strategies used by people with vision impairment, but have relevance to all participants.
- Using a white walking stick or cane for vision impairment. Show the different canes, demonstrating the low-vision ones first. (The long cane and mobility techniques for a blind person are not relevant for the group, but demonstrate the technique briefly.) Often the most appropriate cane is a regular walking stick with light-coloured markings. The presenter can show how to add light and iridescent markings to a cane. We purchased some reflective fluoro Velcro tapes from a specialist bicycle shop for this purpose.
- Wearing light-coloured clothing so as to be seen when out and about, particularly on dull or wintry days.
- Bifocals and multifocals are good for seeing long and short distances at the same time. However, they make step edges, paving edges, kerbs, and stairs inside and outside difficult to see. Be wary and learn to adjust your head position to see better. Indoors, it may be satisfactory to take bifocals off when going up steps or stairs.

Moving around and about

1. When walking, look about six steps ahead to give you time to adjust your steps to potential hazards.
2. When coming from outside to inside, wait till your eyes adjust before coming in. Take sunglasses off when coming inside.

5. Sunglasses and glare. The aim of sunglasses is to protect the eyes from UV rays and to cut down glare. Explain why there are different tints for different needs, and that both a variation in colours and different percentage tints are available. For example, amber or grey colour is thought to be best for use following a cataract operation, and yellow for computer glare. Wrap-around sunglasses (available from Cancer Council shops and often local chemists) that fit over prescription glasses are the most effective. People are generally not aware of the difference that tinting makes. Wearing sunglasses with the tint that works best, rather than the dark sunglasses we all tend to use, gives much clearer vision, and there is a better chance of noticing kerbs and other hazards when moving around outdoors.

Another simple alternative for coping with glare is to wear a hat.

6. Vision services. In addition to regular eye checks by an eye specialist or optometrist, people are generally not aware of the kinds of extra help available to those with vision problems. Many optometrists specialise in low vision. Be aware of local council and health services, specialised low-vision clinics, and services from major vision organisations. The low-vision clinics assist a person in coping functionally with their low vision, rather than fixing the problem. They appear to be a little known and under-utilised facility.

> **An eye specialist can give you eye exercises and low-vision aids to make best use of your vision**
>
> Low-vision clinics and mobility/orientation services may provide mobility aids and, for people with a specific vision condition, may provide assistance with training in their local area.

7. Functional vision at home. If time permits, discuss functional vision inside the home. We usually only touch on major points, such as the lighting options, because the more general issues have been covered in the 'Home fall hazards' session. Let participants know that the handout for today lists some handy hints.

At home

1. Buy the higher lumens light for visibility and cooler day lights for task areas. LED lights are the most cost-effective long-lasting globes and easily available.
2. Clutter can make seeing hazards more difficult. Make sure your hallways, porches and verandas are free from unnecessary items. Don't use thoroughfares as storage areas.
3. Get rid of furniture with castors (like mobile TV stands), or with wide legs (such as table legs) that can stick out and intrude into the walkways where you walk. Get rid of those sausage-shaped draft excluders used to put under doors.
4. Check that there is enough colour contrast between the furniture and the walls and curtains. For example, a white coffee table on a white carpet is easy to trip over.

Night vision

If your vision is worse at night (because, for example, you don't have glasses on), then your balance can be worse. You may also become disorientated in the dark. It is important to use some kind of lighting at night. Photosensitive lights that plug into the power point can help light up a walkway. These can be bought at supermarkets. Touch lamps, bedside lights and torches are a good idea. Install light switches at the top and bottom of stairways.

If glare is a problem:

1. Buy cheap netting or lace curtains to cover windows to shield from the sun in summer.
2. Reduce glare by checking for reflective surfaces and unshielded light bulbs.
3. Halogen lighting gives a bright but diffuse light and can reduce glare.
4. Wear a hat outside and wear sunglasses suitable for your eye condition.

8. Cleaning glasses on a regular basis. If time allows, demonstrate with a soft cloth designed to clean glasses. This reinforces how we can all find it difficult to be aware of poor vision, since we tend to adapt and learn to live with reduced vision. Ask how others clean their glasses and how often.

The break presents an opportunity for participants to ask specific questions of the guest speaker, and for facilitators to reinforce major points during conversations with participants. Brochures can be available for those who want them.

> Remind participants to wear their glasses and have regular check-ups.

Alternative suggestions:

- Encourage people to talk about their functional vision so that they become aware of the effects of any visual decline in their ability to get around in the environment.[1]
- Use glasses that simulate visual problems (e.g. cataracts). Use pathway hazards to demonstrate the effects of reduced vision. This may raise people's awareness of the risks of poor vision and falling. The connection is not always obvious.
- Use large picture cards to demonstrate environmental hazards that can occur in combination with visual impairment, such as slides showing a lack of contrast between furniture, floor, and walls, or situations producing glare.

---

1   See functional vision questions (Clemson, 1997, p. 45).

5.4 GUEST PARTICIPANT TO REFLECT ON THE BARRIERS AND ACHIEVEMENTS TO IMPLEMENTING STEPPING ON STRATEGIES (5 MIN)

Our guest Stepping On graduate was Gerry.

GERRY'S STORY

Gerry came to most of our groups and talked briefly about how the program had helped him. We invited Gerry because he was an articulate and charismatic gentleman. He was perceptive to others' questions and talked gently and openly about his vision. He said that his appearance did not indicate that he had tunnel vision. He described how he took a while to realise his eyesight was poor and how, if he had had the glaucoma diagnosed earlier, it could have been preventable. He has had several falls rushing for the bus. He said that at first he had been cynical because he thought the exercises were too simple, but he found that when he stopped doing them his balance grew worse again. He emphasised that he had learned how important it was to keep doing them. He talked about how he realised he was shuffling as he walked, but that now he goes on long walks, choosing flatter terrain, and making sure that he heel-and-toes and scans ahead. He mentioned how he 'eyeballs the driver'. The footpaths where he lives are old, with big trees. He noticed how he can now lift his feet and step over the cracks. He also spoke about how he had 'slowed down' instead of always rushing. This appeared to spark the interest of the men in the group. His story highlighted positive outcomes of the program, but also showed how he overcame his struggles at different times to keep practising the exercises and to use other safety strategies. The group always listened intently and asked questions.

The facilitator supported our guest participant, as for our other guest speakers, with a phone-call catch-up before the session, prompting Gerry with the topics he planned to talk about. He appreciated this. His agenda was always prepared prior to the group meeting.

5.5   VITAMIN D, CALCIUM AND SUNLIGHT (20 MIN)

This segment is run in a brainstorm and question–answer format. Refer to the 'Topics' section for background information.

Adequate vitamin D and dietary calcium intake has been linked to a reduction in hip fractures. There is also a link to muscle and bone strength, and hence falls and injury prevention. The following outline aims to explore people's knowledge and practices in relation to dietary calcium, and their potential vitamin D status. We explain the relationship between calcium and vitamin D, the consequences of being deficient in either, and how they work in the body.

What does calcium do?

- Calcium increases bone mass (and thus decreases the chance of osteoporosis).
- Calcium is involved in muscle contraction and all of our nerve messages.

Brainstorming activity: What are the sources of calcium?

- Milk, hard cheeses, canned fish with bones, calcium-fortified foods.
- Calcium requirements for women over 50 years and men over 70 years – 1300 mg/day.
- Try to get calcium through your diet.
- If that's not possible, calcium supplements of 500–600 mg can be used. Higher doses should only be used after discussion with a doctor, because of possible side effects.

Homework: Use the 'Calcium checklist for one day' handout to record your daily calcium intake.

What does vitamin D do?

- Vitamin D is essential for the absorption of calcium; together they protect the bones and muscles.
- Vitamin D deficiency has been linked to hip fracture.
- Vitamin D appears to improve muscle quality and protect against bone loss, and may reduce falls.

Brainstorming activity: How do we get vitamin D?

- Sunshine is the main source of vitamin D. Direct sunlight is a good source as it has other benefits. Expose 15 per cent of your body surface (i.e. hands, face, and arms or legs, or an equivalent area of skin) for about 10 minutes in summer and about 20 minutes in winter at least five to six times a week.
- There are limited supplies in certain foods – fatty fish (salmon, tuna, sardines, anchovies), lamb's fry (liver) and eggs – but the foods need to be consumed on a regular basis. Some of our breakfast cereals and milk are fortified with vitamin D, but it is usually in low levels, and these sources are often not a regular part of our diet. Supplements may be needed if participants are not getting enough sunlight.
- The main reason for vitamin D deficiency in older people is limited sun exposure (they don't get out in it enough). Older people don't necessarily need more sun exposure than other people. It is recommended for *all* people that they have periods of sun exposure outside the peak UV periods, i.e. before 10 am and after 2 pm eastern standard time, on most days of the week, exposing 15 per cent of the body surface. (The duration depends on latitude and season.)
- People whose serum levels show a deficiency in vitamin D can take a vitamin D supplement under a doctor's guidance. A maintenance dose of 1000 IU/day is considered sufficient for most people.[2]
- Always get a blood check before taking supplements.

Who is at risk of vitamin D deficiency?

- People who do not get enough sunlight each week, who spend most days indoors because of poor mobility, or who cover up for religious or cultural reasons can suffer bone health problems caused by lack of vitamin D.

How does it work? (Use the poster to demonstrate)

- Vitamin D is formed in the epidermis by the action of sunlight (ultraviolet B rays).
- It is carried by a carrier protein in the bloodstream.
- It is converted into a different form for storage in the liver or activated by the kidneys and the body tissues.

---

2   Duque, Daly, et al., 2017.

- It is then delivered to sites in the body, including muscle, to facilitate calcium and phosphorous absorption (in a process more complex than is understood).

How much sunshine do we need? (Use the poster to demonstrate)

- We need regular, direct sun exposure, not just sunlight coming through a window.
- Expose 15 per cent of your body surface (i.e. hands, face, and arms or legs, or an equivalent area of skin) for about 10 minutes in summer and about 20 minutes in winter, at least five to six times a week.
- Recommended exposure times vary between summer and winter, and according to location (refer to 'Sun time charts' to find the recommended exposure time for a particular locality). For example, in Sydney people need 6–8 minutes in summer and 26–28 minutes in winter, five to six times each week. The times given are one-third of the time it takes to get a faint redness of skin from the sun.
- We recommend going outdoors at least five to six times each week.
- The Cancer Council NSW messages promote covering up, but many people take this to extremes. Just avoid the sun between 10 am and 2 pm (between 11 am and 3 pm during daylight saving).
- Vitamin D deficiency is easily reversible.

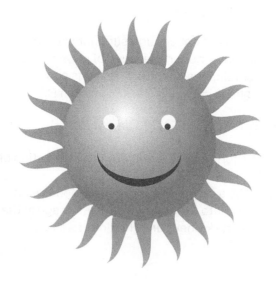

Other benefits of sunshine:

- It makes you feel good!
- There are links between lack of sunlight and depression ('Seasonal Affected Disorder' or 'SAD').
- It encourages regular sleep patterns.

How much sunshine do you get?

- 'Who has been in the sun for x minutes in the past two days? Would you say you get x minutes of sunlight at least three times a week?' If relevant, discuss how the current health messages highlight the dangers of the sun and the risk of skin cancer, which can make us think we should avoid the sun completely. We just need to be sensible when in the sun in some climates.
- Ask: 'How might you increase your sun exposure or vitamin D intake via supplements?'
- Goal setting: 'Check how much sun you get during the next week. Who thinks now that they need to increase the time they spend in the sun?' Hand out the weekly 'Sun time checklist' for those who want to monitor (or try to increase) their sun exposure over the following week. This may indicate whether you are at risk of vitamin D deficiency.

(Hand out the 'Vitamin D and calcium' and 'Sun time checklist' handouts.)

See also:

- Topics: session outline; calcium and vitamin D topic; osteoporosis topic
- Handouts: 'Calcium checklist for one day'; 'Vitamin D and calcium'
- Weekly 'Sun time checklist' for homework.

5.6   TRAVEL SAFETY (15 MIN)

Brainstorming activity: What safety strategies do you use when travelling by bus, train, light rail, or plane?

We do this activity if there is time or else at a later session. Ask participants to brainstorm safety strategies when using bus, light rail, train, or air travel. When the group has exhausted their ideas, add to them, using the travel safety handouts.

To be safe on buses/light rail:

- Be early so you're first in the line.
- Have your money or travel card (Opal, Myki or other) ready.
- Keep a hand free to hold on.
- Take the first seat – up the front if possible.
- Don't get out of your seat or change seats when the bus/light rail is moving.
- Ask the driver to wait until you are seated before setting off.

5.7   HOMEWORK (4 MIN)

Refer to the exercise plan in the 'Balance and strength exercise manual'.

- Determine a personal goal from today's experience. 'Apply something you want to try, and tell the group next week how you went.'
- 'Plan being in the sun for 10–15 minutes about every second day. Take home the "Sun time checklist", and tick off the time spent in the sun during the week.' Remind participants to keep a record of the exercises they do at home.
- Hand out the 'Calcium checklist for one day' handouts and ask people to fill them out for one day next week and then bring them back for discussion.

Vision and falling

People with poor vision are more likely to fall than people with good vision.[1] Half of those people with impaired vision can correct the problem with new glasses.[2]

The following have been significantly associated with falling:[3]

- Poor visual acuity (our ability to see detail such as in signs and reading material). This is tested by the familiar eye charts that most of us have been asked to read at some stage.
- Impaired ability to see contrast sensitivity (our ability to see the edges of borders and objects, or the contrast between light and dark). Loss of edge-contrast sensitivity means that it is difficult to see the edges of objects and paths, and to see obstructions and clutter. Loss of edge-contrast sensitivity is associated with all types of visual loss.
- Poor depth perception or 'stereopsis' (the ability to judge distances and perceive spatial relationships). Depth perception is very important for negotiating obstacles and hazards when walking. It has been found to increase the risk of multiple falls and hip fractures.[4] Having poorer vision in one eye also increases the risk of hip fracture.
- Reduced visual fields; that is, loss of sight in some parts of one's field of view, is a predictor of falls, multiple falls and fractures.[5]
- The presence of cataracts (posterior subscapular cataracts) increases falls. We also know that early removal of cataracts significantly reduces falls.[6]
- People with eye disease (e.g. age-related macular degeneration, glaucoma, and diabetic retinopathy) are at high risk of falls. Macular degeneration is the most common eye disease in older people.[7]
- People who wear glasses with out-of-date prescriptions, or

---

1   Campbell, Reinken, et al., 1981; Ivers, Cumming, et al., 1998; Saftari & Kwon, 2018.
2   Ivers, Cumming, et al., 1998.
3   Ivers, Cumming, et al., 1998; Ivers, Norton, et al., 2000; Lord, Smith, & Menant, 2010.
4   Lord & Dayhew, 2001.
5   Coleman, Cummings, et al., 2007.
6   Gillespie, Robertson, et al., 2012.
7   Ivers, Cumming, et al., 1998.

no glasses, may benefit from new prescriptions. We can be unaware that our vision is slowly changing.

In addition there are other visual difficulties that can affect our ability to negotiate the environment safely:

- loss of central vision in conditions like macular degeneration, and tunnel vision associated with untreated glaucoma
- impaired dark adaptation that can impact spatial orientation at night, or moving between dark and light places
- reduced colour perception, typically related to blues, greens and purples. This indicates that it may be useful to consider halogen, broad-spectrum fluorescent, or warm incandescent lighting to enhance the ability to detect edges and contrast.

Improving illumination at home can improve visual ability. Research has shown that half of the people tested for distance vision and for visual acuity in a clinical situation performed more poorly at home.[8] Visual ability improved with better illumination.

There are useful apps for mobile phones that simulate different eye conditions and demonstrate how people view different environments

WHAT INTERVENTIONS HAVE AND HAVEN'T WORKED?

Expedited cataract surgery significantly reduces the rate of falling, and people should be encouraged to discuss this with their doctor or eye specialist.[9]

Regarding vision screening assessment and provision of new glasses, there have been two trials with mixed results. One study[10] that screened for impaired vision showed a reduction in falls after referral to the person's usual eye care provider, but this did not reach statistical significance. The other study conducted screening and provided new glasses;[11] unfortunately, falls actually increased significantly. The authors concluded that the people with new glasses needed time to adjust to a new prescription, as many had not had a check-up for some time and the prescriptions were often significantly altered. We recommend regular check-ups, but to take particular care with new lenses.

---

8   Cullinan, Silver, et al., 1979.
9   Gillespie, Robertson, et al., 2012; Harwood, Foss, et al., 2005.
10 Day, Fildes, et al., 2002.
11 Cumming, Ivers, et al., 2007.

One intervention aimed to limit the wearing of multifocal glasses by providing single lens glasses for outdoor use.[12] The study was not effective overall, but a subgroup who were more active outdoors did significantly reduce their falls. However, those people who participated in little outdoor activity significantly increased their falls.

HOME SAFETY INTERVENTION

One study of an occupational therapy home safety assessment for older people with severe vision impairment demonstrated a large and significant reduction in falls.[13] This was attributed to the removal and modification of home fall hazards, increased awareness of the environment, and tailored advice from and joint problem-solving with a trained professional. The study showed that exercise alone was not effective in this group as follow-through was low.

VISION AND BALANCE

Our ability to maintain balance is influenced by our multiple motor, sensory, proprioceptive, vestibular and visual systems. How vision dominates this process can be demonstrated when people close their eyes. Postural sway increases by 20–70 per cent.[14] This suggests that balance can be worse at night if vision is worse (e.g. if a person does not have their glasses on or does not have lighting on) and that this can add to the danger of falling.

This is another opportunity to reinforce the importance of the muscle strength and balance exercises for reducing the risk of falling.

VISION AND ENVIRONMENT

People who fall also tend to rely more on visual cues from the environment when mobilising than those who do not fall.[15] The environment needs to maximise visibility, to be uncluttered, and to have safe pathways and walkways. Other considerations would be safe footwear (good fit, support, low heel and non-slip sole) and safety in climbing and reaching.

12   Haran, Cameron, et al., 2010.
13   Campbell, Robertson, et al., 2005.
14   Lord, Smith, & Menant, 2010.
15   Tobis, Reinsch, et al., 1985.

LIGHTING

Lighting considerations depend on the type of eye condition, the environment itself, and the particular circumstances.

- Increase the wattage of the light bulbs used at home. This seems to be the more frequent lighting change needed at home. Enhancing the lighting in dimly lit areas increases visual acuity and the ability to detect contrasts and edges. Increased wattage does not necessarily mean that the electricity bill will be higher (thanks to compact fluorescents).
- If vision is very poor, change to broad-spectrum fluorescent lighting. This gives a more natural lighting and is lighting often preferred by older people. Compact fluorescent light bulbs last around eight times longer than normal bulbs and use up to 80 per cent less energy.
- Make the most of natural light in the home. This may involve structural changes, such as installing a skylight, or be as simple as opening the curtains. Light-coloured walls and furnishings will also enhance illumination, although be sure to maintain some colour contrast between the floor coverings and the furniture.
- Use halogen lighting. This gives a bright but soft lighting and therefore can reduce glare. It is likely to be the most suitable for working in.
- Modify situations that cast shadows.
- If glare is a problem, check for reflective surfaces and unshielded light bulbs.
- Consider your lighting at different times of the day, seasonal variations, and in specific areas such as doorways, step landings, and routes to the bathroom at night.
- Use daylight globes.
- Think of alternative ways to change light globes.

In addition to lighting, the following are some examples of environmental adaptations:

- Avoid clutter. Clutter can make it more difficult to see objects in the way and contribute to trip hazards.
- Be aware of furniture (such as sticking-out table legs and mobile TV stands with castors) that can intrude into the walkways.
- Remember, the eyes may need time to adapt to sudden changes (e.g. coming from outside to inside). Rushing about can contribute to difficulties. It may require concentration to change habits.
- Use colour contrast and safety strips to highlight step edges and changes in level, making them safer.
- Ensure contrast between furniture and walls or curtains.
- When moving about outdoors, scan ahead for hazards. This allows time to adjust one's gait and avoid the hazard. We teach program participants to scan ahead for about four to six steps (about a car length). While it seems obvious, we point out that it may be necessary to look down on reaching the hazard. The distance to scan ahead will depend on the person's vision and their physical capacity to adjust their step to avoid the hazard.
- Be careful of pets. Feed them away from access and walkways.
- Wipe up spills straight away, and remove slippery moss from pathways.

Calcium and vitamin D

Calcium and vitamin D are together the two key ingredients for building and maintaining bone strength and protecting us from fractures.[1] Vitamin D improves muscle strength and reduces the risk of falls.[2]

Calcium crystallises in the bones and gives them their strength and structure. Bones are the calcium bank of the body, storing 99 per cent of our body's calcium. When there is not enough calcium in the diet, other organs and muscles take it from the bones. Over time, this can result in bones becoming thinner and less dense, leading to osteomalacia or osteoporosis and increasing the risk of fracture.

A deficiency of vitamin D is associated with risk of bone loss and fracture in older people, including hip fracture.[3] However, people who are not vitamin D deficient should not take supplements. We recommend natural exposure to sunlight for most people. Calcium absorption is dependent on adequate vitamin D. Vitamin D also appears to have a vital role in the maintenance of muscle strength.

The following is additional background information. We recommend the display include: (i) a 'Calcium content of foods chart', (ii) additional vitamin D information and (iii) osteoporosis information (downloadable sheets are available from Osteoporosis Australia) (see 'Part 3: Resources'). A laminated poster of the pictures of calcium-rich food is useful, as are props such as actual milk containers, cheese packets, etc.

1   Duque, Daly, et al., 2017.
2   Duque, Daly, et al., 2017; Ringe, 2012.
3   Chapuy, Arlot, et al., 1992; Duque, Daly, et al., 2017.

CALCIUM FOOD SOURCES

We start with calcium because more people know about calcium sources and what calcium does, although this does not mean they are consuming adequate amounts.

Calcium requirements increase with age because the body becomes less efficient at absorption. The recommended daily intake of calcium for men older than 70 years and women older than 50 years is 1300 mg of calcium per day. Three serves of dairy products will give most adults their daily needs of calcium.

A 'serve' is 250 mL (8 oz) milk, 200 g yoghurt or two slices of cheese (enough to fit in a matchbox). As a rule, hard cheeses contain more calcium than soft ones, and low-fat dairy products are more concentrated in calcium than higher-fat varieties. Other good sources of calcium are canned fish with bones (salmon, sardines, mackerel or anchovies), almonds and dried apricots.

There are some foods that have been fortified with calcium, which may be an alternative for those who are unable or unwilling to consume dairy products. These foods include some orange juices, breads, cereals and soy milk. Soy products do not necessarily contain calcium unless fortified, so check the product label. The calcium in these products is absorbed equally as well as that in dairy products.

Up to three-quarters of adults do not consume adequate daily calcium. Several forms of supplements are available. Talk to your doctor. Supplements are best utilised by the body at night, so are best taken in the evening.

It is unlikely that too much calcium could be consumed through the diet. Diet is the preferred form of calcium. However, when supplements are given, it is best to aim for a total intake of less than 2000 mg per day, because in some cases overconsumption can increase the risk of kidney stones. For example, if a person gets 800 mg per day from food, then the supplement could be for 800 mg.

Have a calcium content of foods chart on the display table (check the Osteoporosis Australia website) and invite participants to take it home and calculate their average daily intake. If any participants are concerned about their weight, their diet, or their calcium intake, suggest that they ask their medical practitioner for a referral to a dietitian.

VITAMIN D: WHAT DOES IT DO?

Vitamin D is extremely important in protecting against hip and other fractures, and it also plays a role in the maintenance of muscle strength. Vitamin D is necessary for the efficient absorption of dietary calcium and for normal mineralisation of bone. A low vitamin D level in the blood impairs calcium absorption and increases parathyroid hormone production, which can cause bone loss.

An article on the website of the Vitamin D Council[4] describes how vitamin D is converted into different forms, transported and used in the body:

- UVB exposure causes 7-dehydrocholesterol to turn into previtamin D3 in the epidermis.
- This gets 'rearranged' to form vitamin D3, which is bound to a 'binding protein' that carries it all over the body, and to the liver in particular.
- If instead, your intake is in food or as a supplement, it gets absorbed in the small intestine, binds to the same 'binding protein' and transported to the liver.
- In the liver, it gets turned into 'calcidiol' (also called 25(OH)D) for storage and for supplying the body with what it needs. This is the form that should be measured to indicate your level.
- The tissues (and the kidneys) turn the storage form into $1,25(OH)_2D$ (also called 'calcitriol' or 'activated vitamin D'). The activated vitamin D helps all of your body to have the right calcium and phosphorous balance in your blood and tissues. It appears to have other roles as well.

Older women with a vitamin D deficiency are at greater risk of fractures than their peers. According to a French study, half of the women who suffered a broken hip did not have an adequate supply of vitamin D.[5]

Research has shown that taking vitamin D supplements along with calcium will reduce fractures from falls in people who do not have adequate levels of serum vitamin D.[6] A medical physician can test for vitamin D deficiency with a blood test.

---

4   www.vitamindcouncil.org/the-physiology-of-vitamin-d
5   LeBoff, Kohlmeier, et al., 1999.
6   Duque, Daly, et al., 2017.

Vitamin D deficiency is easily reversible. There are two major sources:

1. Vitamin D formed by the action of sunlight on the skin, and
2. Vitamin D from supplements.

> Current recommendations for supplements for people over 70 years with low vitamin D levels suggest supplements of 800–1000 IU per day (or equivalent weekly).

Vitamin D is extremely difficult to obtain from natural food sources because, unlike calcium sources, the Vitamin D-containing foods are not consumed on a regular daily basis.

Because vitamin D is fat-soluble, the body can store it for a period of time. Further research is needed to better understand the storage mechanisms and implications for vitamin D uptake, particularly over the winter months.

To absorb vitamin D, direct sunlight is required, as opposed to light through windows. Sunlight has additional beneficial health outcomes, including an increased alertness. Glass, sunscreen and pollution block the action of the UV light on the skin, which prevents the formation of vitamin D.

It is recommended people be exposed to direct sunlight 5–6 times per week. This can include more than one time on the same day.

In summer, exposure is best at mid-morning or mid-afternoon outside peak UV times – most Australian adults will maintain adequate vitamin D levels during typical day-to-day outdoor activities. When the UV index is above 3 (all states during summer and some states in winter months), sun protection measures should be used if outdoors for more than a few minutes. In winter, longer exposure times are needed, preferably around midday. In autumn or winter in states where the UV index is below 3 for most of the day, sun protection isn't needed.

For example, in Sydney, it is expected that 6–8 minutes in summer and 30 minutes in winter will give the equivalent of 1000 IU of vitamin D3. Exposure times for people with highly pigmented (i.e. darker) skin would be 3–4 times longer.

For the recommended sun exposure to avoid skin damage in Australia, see www.osteoporosis.org.au/vitamin-d

SESSION 05

TOPIC

People who believe they may be deficient in vitamin D or who live in latitudes where there are lengthy winters with limited sunshine may need to get their vitamin D level checked. They can request a blood test from their medical practitioner. Frail older people with low baseline levels of vitamin D (<30 nmol/L) show the highest therapeutic benefit from supplements.[7] An initial higher dose may be recommended to get levels up to normal, then supplements of 700–1000 IU (in the form of a capsule) are recommended to maintain the body's requirements.

WHO IS AT RISK?

- older people who go outdoors infrequently
- those who are housebound
- people who live in hostels or nursing homes
- people with dark skin
- people who cover their skin for cultural or religious reasons
- people with medical or skin conditions preventing sun exposure
- people who live in climates with very cold winters and who do not go outside for long periods.

CAN TOO MUCH BE HARMFUL?

Can too high a dose be harmful? Yes! Though it is a very rare health risk, over time, high daily doses of vitamin D can be dangerous because it is stored in the liver. Overconsumption leads to health problems such as kidney damage and bone deformity. Symptoms are loss of appetite, nausea, weakness, frequent urination, and muscle aches and spasms. The safest approach is to have a blood test for vitamin D deficiency and for a doctor to decide whether vitamin D in capsule form is necessary. Dosages of up to 1000 IU do not exceed safe limits.

Cod liver oil is not advised. This is because, although containing high levels of vitamin D, it also contains high levels of vitamin A, which can become toxic and actually have a detrimental effect on the bones.

Some vitamin and mineral supplements contain a quantity of vitamin D. Even though these are good for helping supplement the body's requirements, they are not at a sufficiently high level to provide all the vitamin D daily needs or to reverse a deficiency.

---

7   Duque, 2017.

OSTEOPOROSIS

Osteoporosis is a condition in which the bones become fragile and as a result can break easily. People who have had a fracture and have osteoporosis have a 50 per cent chance of having another fracture, very often of the wrist, spine or hip.

What are symptoms that could suggest osteoporosis?

- shrinking in height by more than 3 cm (1 inch) due to crushed vertebrae. Two-thirds of spinal fractures go unidentified
- sudden severe and unexplained back pain
- change in posture
- fractures after a minor bump or fall.

Risk factors for osteoporosis include family history of hip fracture, three or more months of corticosteroid treatment, excessive alcohol intake, thin or small body build, and low hormone levels.

Osteoporosis is common, and four out of five people with osteoporosis do not know they have it. Hence, it is often called the silent disease. Anyone over the age of 50 who has had a fracture should discuss having tests for bone mineral density (BMD) and calcium and vitamin D levels with their GP. In Australia, there is a Medicare rebate for BMD tests for people aged over 70 years. Note that heel ultrasounds are not accurate.

A combination of adequate nutrition (vitamin D, calcium and protein) and exercise is important for people with osteoporosis[8] and for protection from falls and fractures.

HOW CAN YOU STRENGTHEN YOUR BONES?

- Get out in the sun to increase your vitamin D level and/or take supplements if deficient – please check with your GP regarding the taking of supplements.
- Get plenty of calcium.
- Avoid smoking.
- Limit your alcohol intake.
- Do regular weight-bearing and resistance exercise.
- Employ fall-prevention strategies.

For further information see www.osteoporosis.org.au

---

8   Daly, 2017.

RECOMMENDED READING

Daly, R. M. (2017). Exercise and nutritional approaches to prevent frail bones, falls and fractures: an update. *Climacteric, 20*(2), 119–124. doi: 10.1080/13697137.2017.1286890

Duque, G., Daly, R. M., Sanders, K., & Kiel, D. P. (2017). Vitamin D, bones and muscle: myth versus reality. *Australasian Journal on Ageing, 36*, 8–13. doi: 10.1111/ajag.12407

Ringe, J. D. (2012). The effect of vitamin D on falls and fractures. *Scandinavian Journal of Clinical and Laboratory Investigation, 72*(S243), 73–78. doi: 10.3109/00365513.2012.681965

Travel safety

Participants brainstorm and discuss helpful hints about safe travel. Choose bus, light rail, train or air safety and do one at a time, depending on group needs. These segments consolidate earlier sections on community safety, drawing on the 'Pedestrian safety' session and the therapist-led 'Moving about safely' segment, and reinforce the importance of the exercises and safe walking. If you do not have time to do all four, save one for another session.

· ·

MAUREEN'S STORY

Maureen had had a bad fall and lost all her confidence in getting about the community. Her son stays with her several days a week and closely oversees her needs. He has helped set up her new house with attractive art and comfortable furniture. She is very committed to the exercises and to scanning ahead and heel-and-toe walking with confidence. She has started to use the buses again, and, against her son's wishes, proudly travels to the city once a week to meet her daughter for lunch. She now plans where to sit on the bus, knows how to get on and off safely, phones when she is nearly there, and her daughter comes to meet her. She says she feels stronger and admits she had been depressed with her situation. She has made new friends in the group and is now going to adult education classes to learn computer skills. She says she enjoys Solitaire and it has helped her to master 'the mouse thing'.

· ·

We limited our mastery experience to one session outdoors and, being a research project, we were restricted by our protocol. Beth Cheal successfully included a mastery experience on buses with her group participants in her 'Steady as You Go' confidence program.[1] If you can arrange it, we recommend including some individual or small-group mobility work including bus or train travel for some participants. It is an excellent way of enhancing people's competence and self-efficacy in coping with travel.

---

1   Cheal & Clemson, 2001.

To develop customised travel-with-safety handouts, we built on our experiences and knowledge, asking the participants in the early groups to brainstorm ideas (which we continue to do), as well as using the internet. Many government transportation departments provide information and helpful hints online. You can continue to update your handouts and provide local knowledge using these strategies.

The following additional information, depending on the needs of the participants, can be used to supplement both the list of strategies that the group brainstorms and the handout.

The following section is dependent upon local travel resources and conditions, and should be adjusted accordingly (see 'Part 3: Resources' for additional local information).

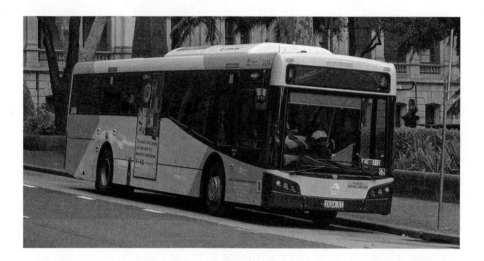

BUS TRAVEL

(Hand out the 'Bus travel safety' handouts.)

Brainstorm strategies for managing buses safely and confidently.

- In some cases, you can plan ahead to use accessible buses. Many accessible buses are equipped to allow passengers to get in and out without a step, and are not intended just for people who use a wheelchair. Ask the bus driver to operate the mechanism if he does not automatically do so.
- In New South Wales, you can ring 131 500 and request a timetable of accessible buses (see 'Part 3: Resources' for contact details for other states). Routes that provide accessible buses are marked on the timetable with the letter 'A'.

- In NSW, people with a vision impairment can obtain a permit that entitles them to free travel on Sydney trains, buses and ferries. Call 02 9224 3589 for further information, and contact your local transport department for other states.

TRAM/LIGHT RAIL TRAVEL

(Hand out 'Tram/light rail travel safety' handouts.)

- Light rail vehicles can approach from either direction and at any time
- Pay attention and stay alert at all times around light rail – they can move quickly and quietly
- Light rail cannot stop quickly
- Be aware of the tracks when wet or frosty – they become slippery
- Use designated crossing points wherever possible
- Always look both ways before crossing at intersections and crossings.

TRAIN TRAVEL

(Hand out 'Train travel safety' handouts.)

- Plan ahead and ring your local transport line (131 500 in NSW) to talk to someone about your needs for getting on and off the train. Travel in the middle of the train as this is where the guard usually is. Ask the guard to help you get onto the train and to help with your bags. Find out in advance whether there are lifts in the station. When you get into the train, always sit on the first level – don't go up or down the stairs on double-decker trains.
- Carry a collapsible walking stick because it indicates to people that your balance is not good and that you are exercising care. They are also more likely to surrender a seat.
- Travel in non-peak hours.
- If you can't read the station information board, speak to the railway staff.
- Some transportation stations have a microphone and amplifier at the ticket office and in some cases by the station information board, to assist hearing-impaired passengers. The station may have other services available to assist people with sensory impairments.
- Anyone who has a disability, which includes you if you use a walking stick or walker, or has difficulty getting on or off the train or subway, can telephone the office before your trip.

One of our participants, John, tested this system for us and found it extremely helpful. Since his stroke he had lived in an apartment on his own. He needed a walking stick and was finding it difficult to get around. He wanted to visit friends, so he contacted the train station and was put through to the destination station. They made appropriate arrangements and were able to help him off the train.

- There may be special features at some stations: lifts or ramps; hearing centres at booking offices or toll booths to make communication easier; continuous handrails; additional lighting; and special signage.
- Take care and take your time.

Facilitators can check local transportation offices for more information for class participants.

AIRLINE TRAVEL

(Hand out 'Airline travel' handouts.)

- Depending on the airline, you can call ahead to make arrangements for hearing assistance, wheelchairs, or other special help. Also available are meals for diabetic passengers, vegetarians, and others with special diets.
- An airline employee may be available to assist passengers on and off the plane. It is wise to call ahead to find out if the service will be available on the day and time of the flight.
- Airports are usually accessible to people with special needs. Escalators, elevators, moving walkways, and baggage carts can be used to make moving through the terminal easier.
- Be sure to make the reservation for your air travel as far in advance as possible, and to ask for any special assistance or accommodations at the time of reservation. You may also want to call and confirm the flight and the assistance you need a day or two before you are scheduled to depart.

Session 6

—

Medication management, sleeping better and mobility mastery experiences

OBJECTIVES

The objectives of this session are to:

1. Understand the importance of having a regular medications review with your doctor or pharmacist.
2. Understand the consequences of taking multiple medications.
3. Understand the consequences of not taking medications in the exact way they are prescribed.
4. Understand the risks of chronic use of sleeping tablets (sedatives).
5. Identify alternatives to improve sleep hygiene.
6. Identify ways of finding out about unwanted effects of medications.
7. Practise mobility situations in a safe and supportive way.
8. Improve confidence in mobility situations when applying safe strategies.

RESOURCES FOR SESSION 6

Session materials: Session 6 agenda; name tags; attendance sheet; display board and display items; flip chart, butcher's paper or whiteboard; marker pen; door signs.

Handouts and flyers: 'Personal medication record cards'; 'Falls prevention and managing medicines', 'Sleeping better'; other relevant community resources and any additional handouts from the speaker.

Catering: snacks and beverages for break.

Other resources: leg weights; audiovisual resources as required by guest speakers.

PREPARING MEDICATION MANAGEMENT EXPERT

Copy topic area 'Medication management', 'Medication management to reduce falls', outline: 'Managing medications' and give a sample of 'Personal medication record card'.

Outline of Session 6: Medication management, sleeping better and mobility mastery experiences

6.1 WELCOME 4 MIN	Welcome and introduction of the guests. Briefly outline today's program. Ask the group for three messages they remember from last week.
6.2 REVIEW OF HOMEWORK 3 MIN	'Did anyone apply anything from the vision and falls segment last week? Do you think having regular eye checks can prevent a fall? How much sunlight did people get during the past week? Has anyone brought in the "Sun time checklist" handout?'
6.3 MEDICATION MANAGEMENT 35 MIN	Guest speaker to lead a participatory-style presentation about medications and falls. Facilitator recaps key points.
6.4 SLEEPING BETTER 20 MIN	Sedatives and falls risk. Behavioural strategies for sleeping better as alternatives to taking medications.
6.5 STRENGTH AND BALANCE EXERCISES 20 MIN	Practise selected exercises with the therapist and invite questions. Advance exercises as able (15 min). Ideas for continuing exercises after the group finishes. Community exercise provider to provide examples of local exercise group (5 mins).
BREAK 15 MIN	
6.6 MOBILITY MASTERY EXPERIENCES 35 MIN	Practise walking over kerbs, kerb ramps, slopes, grassy areas, and steps. During the activity, talk about vision and community safety, and the mobility messages from previous sessions.
6.7 HOMEWORK 4 MIN	'Write up medications on the "Personal medication record card" and, if possible, show it to the pharmacist or doctor. Let us know next week how you managed.' 'Is there anything you particularly want to revise next week in our final session?'

6.1　WELCOME AND OUTLINE (4 MIN)

Welcome participants, introduce speakers and briefly outline the session.

Always ask the group for three things they remember from last week.

6.2　REVIEW THE HOMEWORK (3 MIN)

'Did anyone apply anything from the vision and falls segment last week? Do you think having regular eye checks can prevent a fall?'

'How much sunlight did people get during last week? Has anyone brought in the "Sun time checklist" handout?'

6.3　MEDICATION MANAGEMENT (35 MIN)

(Our guest speaker will complete this section. Hand out the 'Personal medication record cards'.)

You'll need some kind of medical expert for your guest speaker for this segment, preferably a pharmacist who is familiar with medications for the elderly. In your area there may be a pharmacist who is regularly available for consultation about medications through a home visit. Check with a local pharmacy or local doctor regarding this possibility. This is an important session, because research has shown that medication usage can significantly contribute to falls and increase the risk of further falls.

The goals of this segment are to:

1. Demonstrate the risks of medications with respect to falling.
2. Encourage participants to use a 'Personal medication record card' and to show it to their GP, specialist(s) and pharmacist at regular intervals, as well as to other health-care professionals involved in their care. The goal is to make sure that:
    -   When a new medication is prescribed, their doctor(s) and pharmacist are aware of all the medications they are currently taking and therefore possible interactions.
    -   The GP and specialists regularly review the medications so that those that are not needed are ceased, and that dosages are adjusted as needed.
    -   It clearly records how often and exactly how the medications should be taken.
    -   It is comprehensive, accurate and kept current.
3. Identify ways for participants to find out the unwanted effects of medications, and discuss those effects in relation to the risk of falling.

4. Encourage participants to plan ahead before visits to the doctor and to ask questions until an answer is received. We often accept what the doctor tells us without question, but we have a right to be able to understand what we are told and for the important information to be written down. It is not easy for most of us to ask questions, so some time is spent talking about asking questions, how to go about it, its importance, and the kinds of questions to ask.

5. Encourage participants to have a regular pharmacist who will give them information about their medications.

6. Recommend avoiding sleeping tablets, and discuss ways to improve sleep hygiene without the use of medications for sleep.

7. Discuss all the forms medication comes in (e.g. prescription medications, over-the-counter medications, vitamins and minerals, and herbal supplements). Any medications bought without a prescription and for regular use should be discussed with the GP first and then written on their 'Personal medication record cards'.

Occasionally we become aware of participants having unwanted side effects from their medications. For example: Megan said to Maizy, 'You seem rather dozy today.' Maizy replied, 'Yes, I think I had two "sleepers" (sleeping tablets) last night instead of one.' She was clearly not focused and was at risk of falling. She tripped a couple of times that morning and became a negative role model, reinforcing to other members to be wary of sedatives and medications for anxiety in the future. While Maizy did not succeed in stopping the sleeping tablets, she did have the dosage reviewed. We believe the message from that story is a preventive one for many people.

The aim is to warn participants of the dangers of regular sedative use, to raise the group's awareness of other methods of coping with sleep difficulties, of the dangers of not taking medications as prescribed, of unwanted side effects of medications, and to have strategies whereby doctors and pharmacists they see can easily review their medications and dosages. The 'Personal medication record card' is a useful tool for prompting regular review.

The format

This segment needs to be presented in a way that is relevant to the various participants' experiences and routines. It uses both brainstorming (generating a list of ideas) and prompts questions for discussion and sharing. The participants are encouraged to share their personal experiences to help illustrate some of the points. This can be facilitated by the presenters using themselves and their own personal experiences as examples, in addition to the prompts. Each person should have a 'Personal medication record cards'. The following outlines the suggested session format.

PSYCHOTROPIC MEDICATIONS
i.e. medications used to treat depression, anxiety, sleep, and other psychiatric disorders

There is strong evidence that these medications can cause falls.

They can cause many unwanted side effects, including drowsiness (which can persist through to the next day), dizziness, confusion, slowed movements and impaired coordination and balance. Ask your doctor or specialist to review the doses (unwanted effects may be dose-related) and the need for these medications.

SLEEPING MEDICINES: ALTERNATIVE SLEEP STRATEGIES

The occasional sleeping tablet does not present a problem, but when taken for longer than a week they can begin to have alarming side effects, including an increased risk of falls and injuries due to falling. Once in a routine or habit, it is extremely difficult to stop taking them, because they cause dependence. Discontinuation of most medications prescribed for sleep problems should be done gradually under a doctor's direction. We recommend using alternative strategies to help you avoid taking sleeping tablets on a regular basis. There is some evidence to suggest that the risk of a fall is highest soon after starting to use them. We will cover sleep alternatives later in the morning (see the 'Topic' section and handout for 'Sleeping better').

MULTIPLE MEDICATIONS

The use of regular multiple medications can increase the risk of interactions, leading to unwanted side effects such as a greater risk of falls. By being aware of this, you can take more care when doing things, or take action to prevent accompanying unwanted side effects such as those listed below.

The 'Personal medication record card'

WHAT IS IT?	Your personal, up-to-date record of all the medicines you are taking – when you started them, what they are for, how and when to take them, and any warnings or advice.
WHY USE IT?	Taking multiple medications may result in a greater risk of falls. Your GP does not always know what other health professionals have prescribed for you. Also, your GP's record of the medications you take may not match what you are actually taking. The 'Personal medication record card' helps you, your pharmacist, and your prescribers better manage your medications. This can prevent some falls.
HOW TO USE IT?	You can ask your GP or pharmacist to update it for you. Include all the prescription medications, over-the-counter medications, vitamin and mineral supplements, and herbal medications you take. Carry the card with you at all times and show it to your doctor at each visit. Ask your GP to review all your medications at least once a year. Show the card to your pharmacist as you ask for information about a new prescription. This will assist in identifying any issues.

Medications and their unwanted side effects

Finding out about your medications and their unwanted side effects is important. You have the right to know and to ask questions. It is your body.

Brainstorming activity: What are some unwanted side effects that could cause a fall?

Once the group have exhausted their ideas, contribute some more from the list below:

- being unsteady on your feet or having poor balance
- having weak muscles or general weakness
- being slower to move about
- being slower to react to a trip or a slip
- feeling confused; finding it harder to think clearly
- having memory problems
- having impaired coordination (mentally or physically)
- having blurred or double vision

- feeling dizzy, light-headed or faint
- being drowsy or tired (e.g. due to unwanted side effect, impaired sleep or over-sedation)
- having impaired alertness
- having a sudden drop in blood pressure

What is the best way to communicate with your doctor?

Before your visit, write a list of what you want to say and what questions to ask. This is a good routine for people of all ages; we can forget at the time all the things we wanted to ask – it is hard to remember everything. 'Has anyone tried making a list? How did it work?'

Don't leave the consultation until you understand what has been said to you. A good marker of understanding is when you can describe the problem and the treatment in your own words. Ask the doctor to clarify the information provided. Ask for the important points to be written down.

Get to know a good pharmacist and stick with them

'Why is this a good idea? What can a pharmacist offer?'

Many pharmacists will offer their time to help you understand unwanted side effects and how to take your medications. They can get to know you and your needs. The pharmacist can be the most important person in helping you manage your medications safely.

Brainstorming activity: What questions about my medicines should I ask my doctor and/or pharmacist?

- What is the medicine for?
- What does it do? What results can I expect?
- Will this medicine interact with other medicines I am taking? Do I need to avoid any other medicines, foods or drinks when I am taking this medicine?
- How should I take my medicine? With water or food?
- When should I take my medicine and for how long?
- What should I do if I miss a dose?
- What are the possible unwanted side effects?
- What should I do if an unwanted side effect occurs? What can I do to manage or lessen the unwanted side effects?
- Do I need regular check-ups or tests while taking this medicine?

- When should it be stopped, or when is the next time to review this medicine?
- Do I still need the same dose?
- What can I do to make it easier for me to take this medicine? (e.g. use a 'blister' pack, Dosette® box, or easy-to-open bottle)
- How should I store this medicine?

Brainstorming activity: What can I do to manage my medications safely?

Once the group have exhausted their ideas, suggest some others from this list:

- Take reasonable care to reduce the effects of known unwanted side effects.
- Know when, how, and how much medication to take – and stick to it.
- If you take several medications, either a Dose Administration Aid such as a 'pill' box, or (preferably) a 'blister' pack prepared by your pharmacist, may be helpful.
- Avoid foods, alcohol and medications (including vitamin supplements and herbal preparations) that can interact with your medications.
- Don't take someone else's medication. It might have a very different effect on your body.
- Start taking the new medication or the higher dosage when you know you are not going to be busy, perhaps on the weekend. If you live alone, start it when you know someone is likely to be around. When you're going on holidays, don't leave it till the last minute to change your medication or start a new medication. Give yourself time to adjust to the changes in your body well before you leave.
- When you get up out of bed, move slowly and pause before you get up. Pause again before you walk off. This may also be a useful strategy when you get out of a chair or in other situations, such as getting out of a car or off the bus.
- If you have been taking a medication over a long period of time, make sure the dose and indication are regularly reviewed by your GP or specialist, even if the dose is always the same. You may find that as you age, a lower dose may be indicated. Other options for review are:
  - asking your GP for a Home Medicines Review (HMR) referral. This is available once every two years. An HMR is an independent review of your medications and management. There is no cost and it is conducted in your home by a pharmacist on referral from your GP.

- – making an appointment with your pharmacist for an in-pharmacy MedsCheck, available once every 12 months. A MedsCheck provides an opportunity to ask about unwanted side effects and increased risk of falling.
- If you have a fall, always report it to your GP, and check with your GP or pharmacist whether your medications may have contributed to or been the cause of the fall. Be sure to also consider the unwanted side effects of medications *after* having a fall (e.g. bleeding risks if taking a blood thinner; fracture risks).
- Talk to your doctor, specialist or pharmacist about managing certain conditions (e.g. sleep problems) without medications.

Additional brainstorming activity: When a health professional asks what medications you take, what does that include?

Prescription medications, tablets, sprays, patches, herbal products, over-the-counter products, vitamin and mineral supplements, creams, suppositories, pessaries, inhalers, injections, eyedrops, eardrops, anything you take or use.

Note, garlic tablets are considered a medication, whereas eating garlic is not.

> The homework for next week will be to use the 'Personal medication record card'. Remember to include all forms of medications you use. Encourage participants who have the opportunity to see a doctor or pharmacist during the week to ask at the appointment for a review of their medication list and report back to the group the next week.

Alternative suggestions:

- Role play: asking a pharmacist questions about your new prescription
- Role play: asking a doctor or pharmacist to review all your medications.

6.4 SLEEPING BETTER (20 MIN)

This segment explains the link between sedatives and falls. Behavioural strategies that are known to help people sleep better are offered as alternatives to taking medications on a regular basis.

Sleep problems are not due to ageing, but can be genetic, physical or psychological, or can develop because of things we do. There is normally a reason for having a sleep problem. As we age, we experience less of the deeper rapid eye movement (REM) sleep and more of the lighter (non-REM) sleep. This is natural. But insomnia is NOT a result of ageing – so if it is persistent, discuss it with a doctor. In addition, now we know there is a lot we can do *ourselves* to help us sleep better.

See Session 6 'Topics' section for background information to help guide the questions and answers. The behavioural strategies are summarised in the handout 'Sleeping better'. The major part of this session is a brainstorming activity generating solutions to sleeping better. The following outlines the key points for discussion and the brainstorming activities for this session.

Sleeping pills – not good to take over a long time:

- Sleeping pills are acceptable for a time of crisis or on occasion when needed, but have no real demonstrated effect on insomnia. It is best not to start taking them on a regular basis.
- There are some other approaches that can help with sleep problems.
- If taking sedatives on a regular basis, try reducing the dose slowly under a doctor's supervision.

The side effects of taking sleeping pills for a long time can include:

- daytime hangover effects
- daytime sleepiness
- falls and confusion
- more sleep problems
- addiction.

Brainstorming activity: Who sleeps well at night? What are the things that we can do to help us have a good night's sleep?

Write participants' answers on a flip chart or whiteboard. Once they finish brainstorming their solutions, ask them:

Do you need to sleep more as you get older?

A good quality sleep does not mean that we have to have longer sleep, and actually as we age we need less of the deep sleep. We experience less of the deeper REM sleep and more of the lighter (non-REM) sleep. This is natural. But sleep disturbances are not a natural part of ageing.

Naps are good, but don't have them for more than 20 minutes or so.

Now pass around the 'Sleeping better' handouts. Be sure to praise the group for the many points they generated and identify ones they might have missed.

There can be many underlying reasons why we do not sleep, and if people have persistent sleeping disturbances, they should see their doctor to diagnose the causes. Insomnia and sleep apnoea can be diagnosed.[1]

Alternative activity: Mrs Charles has been having falls and has been experiencing some of the unwanted side effects mentioned above. She has realised this relates to taking sleeping tablets. She is now thinking about what stops her sleeping at night and what she can do to fix this.

Participants are given a prop with an accompanying card that has a large-print statement that they share with the group. For example, a crazy clock accompanies: 'I keep checking the time at night when I can't sleep', a large novelty mug accompanies: 'I like my coffee and scotch just before I go to bed.' Do you think these things would help or hinder? What works for you?

6.5 STRENGTH AND BALANCE EXERCISES (20 MIN)

(Another guest speaker will complete this section – a therapist.)

Practise the exercises with the physiotherapist and invite questions. Explain the need to increase weights and upgrade the balance exercises.

Consider providing a fridge magnet of the exercises as a prompt (see handouts for a copy that can be reproduced as a fridge magnet).

Invite a local exercise provider to come and share their program and how to access it when Stepping On finishes. Ensure the program fits and has the right balance and strength exercises for fall prevention.

A past participant can also be invited to talk about the benefits of exercise for them and also the challenges of relapse – how to keep it going.

1   See Rodriguez, Dzierzewski, & Alessi, 2015 for screening check lists.

Display leaflets and information on local community fall groups and also community transport options.

6.6   MOBILITY MASTERY EXPERIENCES (35 MIN)

The purpose of this segment is to provide an opportunity for participants to put into practice, and gain some mastery over, some of their personal mobility goals. It provides a supportive environment in which to practise those goals, with assistance as needed and instruction on technique. In this segment, we take the group outdoors to practise mastery of safe strategies for steps, uneven ground, kerbs, etc. So check the most suitable outdoor space at or near your venue, because you will not have time to go far. If you are unable to go outside, practise inside and do a demonstration with some steps, or obstacles to walk around, to simulate outdoors. We have found it best to go outdoors if possible. The participants usually have a range of mobility needs: there are those people who are more active and not as interested in the detail and the slow pace of the mobility mastery experiences, and those who have mobility difficulties. We pitch these two segments at different levels.

Community mobility mastery experiences for those who have mobility difficulties

Example: Meg uses a walking stick if she is walking outside for any distance. She has a spinal curvature and, at the beginning of the program, was extremely weak. She revealed how sceptical she had been about the exercises and the program at the beginning. She is a retired physical therapist and found it difficult to be the recipient of a health program. She said it took her seven weeks to realise some benefits and accept the idea, which is our experience with many of our participants. She found this session was particularly useful for trying out kerbs and inclines in the company of someone who could provide feedback and support.

This session requires considerable pre-planning. It is useful to have extra helpers to partner the participants, which maximises the opportunity to discuss issues while the activity is being performed. We try to get our therapist along for the exercise session just before break time (to answer any questions about the exercises) and then to stay for the mobility mastery session. Their expertise and input are invaluable.

Be creative about where you can find the most suitable venue. Think about what it offers that your particular group needs. There may be useful features as close as just outside the front of your venue, or a little way down the road, or you may be near a local park or shopping centre.

Discussion and the mobility goal setting indicated that our particular group was worried about:

1. uneven footpaths
2. uneven ground
3. hurrying and not paying attention
4. steps and stairs
5. standing up and feeling giddy.

We go out to the front of our venue and can usually find most of the following: steps with and without handrails, uneven ground, different surfaces (grass, gravel) and a variety of different gradients, kerbs and steps. People often feel most anxious on the downhill slope: they practise using a wider gait to walk there, and sometimes decide they would plan to be very careful or avoid such slopes.

The format of the master mobility session

Get the mastery subgroup together before setting out. Explain the intended aims and check any special requests. Explain that we are going to put into practice some of the things we have learned, such as scanning ahead and going up steps (choose the most appropriate from the practice list below).

'This is an opportunity, now that you have been improving your balance and strength, to see that situations you once found challenging are now much easier to manage. It is also a chance to reflect on how we normally do things as we get out and about. It's a way of connecting the theory and the practice, and to see how we apply some of these things in different circumstances.'

Explain where you are going and what the opportunities are.

For example: 'As we leave the building, there are steps with a handrail and a ramp. When we get to the park, etc.'

Along with the other staff, 'buddy up' with a participant or a couple of participants. As you walk along with the participant, talk about what is being practised, encouraging the older person to share things from the program that they have tried out, and prompting safe techniques if necessary. This section brings together strategies taught in all the previous sessions, including the community mobility and vision segments.

Try to include a planning exercise: 'If we had to cross the road, where would the safest place be, and what is the best way for us to do it?'

If participants do not seem to be concentrating on anything in particular, or if they finish with what they are keen to try out, then prompt to facilitate further observations. It is best to respond to what participants need rather than attempting to cover everything. Prompt with comments that may help them to think. For example: 'Do you think you are wearing safe shoes for this sort of situation? Are you climbing with the stronger leg upwards first? How do you feel about getting out and doing the shopping? How do you actually do your shopping? Have you noticed the timing of the lights, and do you feel you are more confident crossing the street at the lights now?

Refer questions to the therapist when in doubt. The therapist can move to different people as needed (e.g. for handling steps and kerbs) and as questions arise.

Practise as many of the following as you can. Copy and enlarge this list to give it to any extra helpers, so they can be ready for a purposeful chat with their partner(s).

The following is a useful summary that can also be given as a handout

Walking outside:

- Scan ahead when walking. It helps you to be prepared when approaching hazards and gives you time to adjust your step to avoid the hazard. 'Have you tried this? How did you do it? How far do you scan? What works best? Why do we scan ahead?'
- Practise heel-and-toe walking
- Adjust to different surfaces
- Use shoes for outdoors

Steps:

- Decide which leg down first? Which leg up first?
- Walk one step at a time, if need be
- Use handrails
- Mark the edges of steps with brightly coloured tape
- Use elevators, when available, instead of stairs

Walking up a slope:

- Walk with feet farther apart
- Take smaller steps

- Use a cane or walking stick
- When walking on ramps, use handrails

Different surfaces:

- Scan ahead when walking
- Look out for change from carpeting to linoleum, hardwood floors, or tiles. How do you clear the thresholds? How do you change your step?
- On slippery surfaces, walk with feet wider apart or take smaller steps; use a cane or walking stick; put traction on shoes or boots. Plan ahead to avoid slippery surfaces like wet spills or ice.
- Grass can be slippery, especially if wet; it can hide uneven spots or holes, and it can be high and catch your toes. Use heel-and-toe walking and a wider base over grass. Point out how this also improves the strength of ankles. 'If you know you are going over grass that may be wet, what shoes would it be best to wear? Plan the best route to take.'
- On uneven ground or footpaths, practise heel-and-toe walking, adjust steps, and/or use a walking stick or cane.
- If you are unable to practise outdoors, you can use doormats with different surfaces – for example, a mat with high bristles.

Crossing a road:

- Plan the safest and best way to cross the road. 'What do you look for and what do you try to avoid?'
- 'Eyeball' the drivers before crossing the road
- Don't rush
- Cross with the light using the pedestrian crossing
- Cross with a group of people
- Remember not to cross between parked cars
- Go out when it is not peak hour
- Wear your hearing aid to hear car horns and engine sounds
- Climb a kerb
- Plan the best spot to use. Is there a pole to hold onto? What else could you use (e.g. a walking stick or the arm of a friend)?
- Think which foot goes up first? Which foot goes down first?

Vision:

- Does anyone wear bifocals or multifocals? What kinds of difficulties do you encounter? How do you get around these? Do you take off your glasses when negotiating steps or have you learned to adjust your head position to see?

- Check light conditions
- Wear sunglasses (refer to the vision presentation in Session 4). Ask: 'How do sunglasses help?' Discuss glare.
- Plan ahead when you leave home
- Leave the outside lights on or use motion lights
- Carry a flashlight or torch
- Park under a street light
- When going into different lighting (for example, from light to dark), stop until your eyes adjust. Use a cane or walking aid.
- Wear white at night so drivers can see you.

Windy days:

- Talk about managing on windy days.
- Wear a back pack so your hands are free.
- Use community transport on a windy or rainy day. Windy days are perhaps best avoided for some people.

Snow or ice:

- Scan ahead for ice or frost
- Wear shoes or boots with more tread
- Wear Yaktrax®
- Walk slower and with smaller steps
- Practise heel-and-toe walking
- Raise awareness of community services, e.g. a community bus
- Provide information about local community transport options.

Review as a group what they have achieved and whether they met any of their personal goals. What strategies did people try, e.g. defensive walking and scanning ahead?

Example: One group went to a nearby shopping complex. Most found uneven ground, ramps, crowds, and their own poor eyesight the most difficult things to cope with. Several people reported they used the shopping carts to create space around them as a way of saying, 'Keep your distance!' to other people.

6.7 HOMEWORK AND PLANNING NEXT WEEK (4 MIN)

Briefly recap the main points from the medication talk and community mobility.

Homework: Fill out the 'Personal medication record card'. If anyone is going to the doctor or can see their pharmacist, ask them to fill out the 'Personal medication record card' and to let the group know next week how it went.

Question: 'Is there anything you particularly want to revisit next week in our final weekly session?'

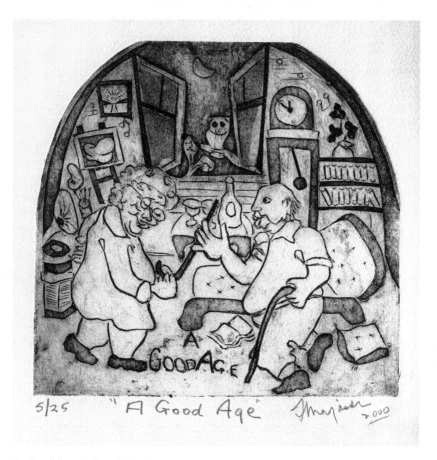

"A Good Age" by Frank Marjason.

Medication management to reduce falls

Older people tend to be more sensitive to both the intended (therapeutic) and adverse effects of medications. Polypharmacy to address comorbidities is also more common in older people, and this may cause undesirable drug interactions. Although many medication classes have been linked to falls, the evidence is strongest for psychotropic medications and other medications with effects on the central nervous system and cardiovascular system.

Many medications can increase the risk of falls through various mechanisms, such as:

- sedation due to psychotropics (such as sleeping tablets, antidepressants, antipsychotics), sedating antihistamines, opioids, etc.
- impaired cognition due to psychotropics, anticholinergics, opioids, etc.
- hypotension (low blood pressure) due to cardiovascular drugs, antidepressants, antipsychotics, opioids, Parkinson's medications, etc.
- anticholinergic adverse effects such as dizziness, blurred vision and confusion due to some antidepressants, urinary incontinence medications, antihistamines, opioids, antipsychotics, COPD medications, Parkinson's medications, etc.

The use of multiple medications may have additive unwanted side effects, resulting in an increased risk of falls. As described above, there are many medications that can cause hypotension, including postural hypotension, which causes dizziness when you stand up (often, hypotensive effects are dose-related). There are also many medications used for many different indications with sedative and/or anticholinergic effects, which are cumulative. The use of multiple medications may also result in increased interactions between drugs and increased risk of incorrect use of medications.

Reviews with a GP are recommended annually, or more often if there has been a visit to hospital or an event such as a fall has occurred. Other options for medication review are:

- asking the GP for a Home Medicines Review (HMR), which is a collaborative process undertaken with an accredited pharmacist, in the patient's home, available once every two years
- making an appointment with the community pharmacist for a MedsCheck, available once every 12 months.

Being aware of potential unwanted side effects of medications and ensuring regular reviews of medications are reasonable strategies to help reduce the risk of falls when taking multiple medications. It is advisable for participants to make an appointment with a pharmacist for a review of their personal list of medications to identify known unwanted side effects. We recommend participants keep a 'Personal medication record card' up-to-date and take it with them whenever they see their GP, specialist or other health professionals involved in their care.

EVIDENCE FROM RESEARCH

- Physician-prescribed withdrawal of medications associated with falls risk can reduce falls by up to 66 per cent.[1]
- A medication review to improve the use of medicines reduced falls by up to 39 per cent.[2]
- There is a significant increase in risk of falls when taking sedatives, antidepressants or benzodiazepines.[3]
- Sleeping tablets should never be used on a regular basis. The side effects of taking sleeping tablets for more than a week include daytime hangover effects, confusion and daytime sleepiness, a risk of falling, and more sleep problems. Tolerance to the hypnotic effects of sleeping tablets occurs within weeks (i.e. they no longer help you get to sleep).
- Antidepressants result in sedation, leading to psychomotor retardation (slower walking speed), impaired balance, and frequently postural hypotension, and these are probably the main reasons that they can cause falls.
- Antipsychotics can result in sedation and slowing of motor function, gait disturbances (extrapyramidal), related visual blurring (anticholinergic), and (in some cases) cataracts and other visual problems.

1   Campbell, Robertson, et al., 1999; van der Velde, Stricker, et al., 2007.
2   Pit, Byles, et al., 2007.
3   Woolcott, Richardson, et al., 2009.

- There is a significant increase in fall-related hospitalisation (up to 1.5-fold) when taking five or more medicines with anticholinergic and sedative effects.[4]
- There is an increase of over 20 per cent of serious fall injuries over five years with antihypertensive use.[5]
- Cardiovascular medications account for approximately one-third of adverse drug reactions, symptoms and signs that are also fall risk factors (e.g. weakness, dizziness, poor balance, fatigue). There is a 30 per cent risk of falls associated with medicines in patients taking antihypertensive medications, compared with 10 per cent for those not taking antihypertensives.[6]
- If you are taking blood-thinning medications (known as anticoagulants), monitor your bleeding risks especially after falling or being injured from a fall, remembering to report the fall to your GP.

RECOMMENDED READING

Boyle, N., Naganathan, V., & Cumming, R. G. (2010). Medication and falls: risk and optimization. *Clinics in Geriatric Medicine, 26*(4), 583–605. doi: 10.1016/j.cger.2010.06

Hill, K. D., & Wee, R. (2012). Psychotropic drug-induced falls in older people. *Drugs & Aging, 29*(1), 15–30. doi: 10.2165/11598420-000000000-00000

Huang, A. R., Mallet, L., Rochefort, C. M., Eguale, T., Buckeridge, D. L., & Tamblyn, R. (2012). Medication-related falls in the elderly. *Drugs & Aging, 29*(5), 359–376. doi: 10.2165/11599460-000000000-00000

---

4   Nishtala, Narayan, et al., 2014.
5   Tinetti, McAvay, et al., 2008.
6   Tinetti, McAvay, et al., 2008.

Sleeping better

A major message for this segment is 'Avoid taking sedatives on a regular basis', and it aims to reach those people in the program who are not regular users. Instead of taking sleeping tablets to alleviate sleep problems, people can be encouraged to try more practical approaches. The aim is prevention.

For many people, ageing brings a natural reduction in Stages 3 and 4 (deep) sleep and a corresponding increase in Stage 1 (light) sleep. This can result in a lighter and sometimes more transitory sleep, which can be wrongly interpreted as a sleep difficulty.[1] Older people often also have an earlier bedtime and an earlier wake time, due to changes to the circadian rhythm. Insomnia (i.e. sleep disturbance) is not an inevitable consequence of ageing. About 50 per cent of people never experience problems sleeping. The others can have difficulty falling asleep or maintaining sleep, or may wake early in the morning, or a combination of these.

REASONS FOR NOT SLEEPING

The reasons for poor sleep can be varied. Sleep problems may be due to a general decline in physical activity, which is a potentially reversible factor. Inactivity, along with decreased light exposure, has been shown to decrease arousal thresholds, elevate autonomic activity, and lead to circadian rhythm changes, all of which can impact on the quantity and quality of sleep. The natural light–dark cycle affects our 24-hour clock. Exposure to natural light (direct or indirect) for at least 30 minutes (and preferably up to two hours) daily is recommended.

In addition, if a person is housebound or socially isolated, a lack of time cues can impact on arousal and sleep patterns. This issue can be addressed. If the sleep disorder is diagnosed as due to sleep apnoea, or sleep-disordered breathing, this condition can be treated. Nocturnal awakening can be for a range of reasons (e.g. gastroesophageal reflux, nocturia, leg cramps) and often results in an increase in daytime sleepiness and napping. Or it may be due to something as simple as a mug of coffee. Caffeine can increase the number of times a person wakes and thus reduces the total sleep time. The range of reasons[2] is summarised below:

---

1   Rodriguez, Dzierzewski, et al., 2015.
2   Cistulli & Singh, 2000; Rodriguez, Dzierzewski, et al., 2015.

- overweight, sleep-disordered breathing
- inactivity, reduced social activity
- reduced natural light exposure, lack of environmental time cues
- pain
- polypharmacy
- sleeping tablets (side effects)
- caffeine
- fluid excretion
- stress
- depression
- alcohol, increased alertness
- respiratory or cardiac conditions
- sleep apnoea (diagnosed)

There may be underlying reasons among these that need attention.

There are some myths about ways to sleep better. False beliefs include:

- Everyone needs 8 hours sleep a night.
- Staying in bed longer and trying harder to sleep will help you sleep better.
- A daytime nap will help you cope with poor night-time sleep.
- Sleeping tablets will give good quality sleep and be effective over a long time.

WHAT APPROACHES TO SLEEPING BETTER ARE EFFECTIVE?

Rodriguez et al.[3] provide an excellent summary of the kinds of approaches that are effective. The 'Sleeping better' handout summarises the most up-to-date approaches that individuals can take to improving their sleep hygiene.

Sedatives are a major risk factor for falls. There are a variety of medications that can cause insomnia in older people, including the long-term use of sedatives. There is less use of these drugs now. If someone is taking sedatives, they should not be stopped abruptly. Research indicates that it is very difficult to get people to cease taking sleeping tablets.[4] It may be useful to review the dosage and reduce it slowly, and to check with the GP or pharmacist that they are being taken as directed and at the correct dose.

---

3   Rodriguez, Dzierzewski, et al., 2015.
4   Campbell, Robertson, et al., 1999.

There is considerable support for the use of behavioural approaches – modifying practices that inhibit good sleeping patterns. Having a consistent sleep schedule, sleep restriction, increased physical activity, and healthy sleep practices (such as bedtime rituals, calming routines and avoiding stimulants before bedtime) can be valuable strategies for improving sleep quality and duration.

Some people will need to give attention to techniques like imagery or relaxation that will help them to cope with anxieties and worries. A study employing mindfulness meditation,[5] using an accessible program (see below), showed immediate improvement in sleep quality in older people.

There is strong evidence that limiting the amount of time spent awake in bed helps – bed is for sleep and sex, not for lying awake in. This is linked to the theory that some people begin to associate bedtime with wakefulness rather than sleeping. It may be better to get out of bed on waking up during the night and to do some quiet activity like reading.

One strategy that might work for some people is to reduce the time in bed each night by half to one hour. A short daytime nap is allowable, but this should be only about 15–30 minutes, and no longer than 45 minutes. Sleep restriction has been shown to improve sleep quality and to give an improved sense of wellbeing during the daytime.[6]

A number of our participants reported that their leg cramps were relieved when they started doing the calf raises exercise. Movement is recommended when restless legs are experienced.

It seems that multicomponent approaches are best, and that these are tailored to the circumstances of the person.[7] The session can be used to encourage discussion about the participants' beliefs about and attitudes to sleeping better, and to initiate problem-solving.

5   Black, O'Reilly, et al., 2015.
6   Hoch, Reynolds, et al., 2001.
7   Morin, Mimeault, & Gagne, 1999.

RESOURCES

(We suggest you include this information on your resources table.)

Mindfulness courses:

- www.sane.org
- www.futurelearn.com/courses/
  mindfulness-wellbeing-performance

Online information on sleeping better:

- Sleeping well (Fact sheet 7) at www.beyondblue.org.au/
  get-support/staying-well/sleeping-well
- 'Sleep tips for older adults' at www.helpguide.org/articles/
  sleep/how-to-sleep-well-as-you-age.htm

RECOMMENDED READING

Rodriguez, J. C., Dzierzewski, J. M., & Alessi, C. A. (2015). Sleep problems in the elderly. *Medical Clinics of North America, 99*(2), 431–439. doi: 10.1016/j. mcna.2014.11.013

Cistulli, P. A., & Singh, N. A. (2000). Sleep. In M. A. Fiatarone Singh (Ed.), *Exercise, nutrition, and the older woman: wellness for women over fifty* (pp. 417–441). London: CRC Press.

SESSION 06

TOPIC

Session 7
—
Reviewing and planning ahead

OBJECTIVES

The objectives of this session are:

1. to acknowledge personal accomplishments
2. to identify the scope of participants' knowledge of falls prevention and to determine attitudes to coping with falling
3. to complete any topics not yet addressed. These usually include strategies to assist in safe use of transportation
4. to offer time for farewells and inform participants of planned follow-up activities.

RESOURCES FOR SESSION 7

Session materials: Session 7 agenda; name tags; attendance sheet; door signs; evaluation forms if needed; graduation certificates.

Handouts: 'Maintaining the momentum after Stepping On'; 'Graduation certificate'.

Catering: snacks and beverages for break, apples for Apple Game.

Other resources: leg weights, Stepping On class follow-up activities – prepare cards with date and time as a reminder.

Outline of Session 7: Reviewing and planning ahead

7.1 OVERVIEW OF TODAY'S SESSION 4 MIN	Welcome participants. Give a brief introduction to the session. Ask the group for three messages they remember from last week.
7.2 REVIEW OF HOMEWORK 5 MIN	'Did anyone fill out the "Personal medication record card"? Did anyone have a chance to review the "Personal medication record card" with a doctor or pharmacist?' 'What about any of the points we covered in "Getting about in the community"? Did anyone try out anything during the week?'

7.3 EXERCISES **8 MIN**	Exercises: 'Last chance to practise selected exercises. Why is strength important? Does anyone need to upgrade the weights?' Advance exercises as able. Discussion of 'How to keep it going'.
7.4 REVISION **35 MIN**	Fall scenario – identify causes and solutions together. And/or play the Apple Game, using questions based on all the major themes. Select questions to recap major themes. Address the following topics if of interest to the group and not already covered: dizziness, travel.

BREAK 15 MIN

7.5 GROUP EVALUATION **35 MIN**	Brainstorming activity: What causes someone to fall? Compare answers to those in the list generated in Session 1. Ask each member: 'What is the major thing you have gained from the program over the last seven weeks?' Have your co-facilitator write down the comments. Conclude with a general group question: 'Do you think falls can be prevented?'
7.6 FAREWELLS AND FOLLOW-UP **10 MIN**	Conclude with the graduation certificates. Very important: Thank everyone for being part of the program. Inform the group of the follow-up activities. Let them know you will send a letter to their doctor saying they completed the program. Invite them to the three-month booster session.

7.1 OVERVIEW OF TODAY (4 MIN)

Always ask the group for three things that they remember from last week.

Today is a time for review, completing what we haven't yet covered, finding what we've got out of the program so far and planning for the future (home visits, phone calls or get-togethers in a few months' time to see participants' progress).

7.2 REVIEW OF HOMEWORK (5 MIN)

'Did anyone fill out the "Personal medication record card"? Did anyone have a chance to review the "Personal medication record card" with a doctor or pharmacist? What about any of the points we covered in "Getting about in the community"? Anyone try out anything during the week?'

7.3 EXERCISES (8 MIN)

Discuss how to continue exercise as part of a regular commitment. Check if anyone wants to upgrade or has purchased extra weights. Discuss on-going exercise classes available in the community. Give out the 'Maintaining the momentum after Stepping On' handout.

7.4 REVISION (35 MIN)

Give out the 'Safety on public transportation' handout.

Fall scenario and discussion

A fall scenario or critical incident generates insights and demonstrates people's problem-solving abilities. Mrs Jardine and the night fall[1] (see Session 1) is a good one if not already used.

Question: What factors do you think could have contributed to her fall?

Answer: Incontinence problems; using a bath instead of a shower; having cataracts and therefore poor night vision; no night-light; not understanding she needed a light at night; relying on her memory rather than strategies that would automatically work; she didn't want to turn on the light because it would be too bright and wake her up too much.

Question: What could she now do to be safer at home and feel more confident?

---

1   Clemson, 1997.

Answer: Have a consistent and safe lighting procedure for night-time. Use an automatic light source that gives a soft light (e.g. a photosensitive night-light). See someone about her cataracts. Investigate the incontinence problems. Review late-night fluid intake. Keep doing her strength and balance exercises so that she might be able to prevent a fall or recover more easily from a fall.

Participants are not expected to come up with all these answers. Rather, it is the discussion and the problem-solving process that is important.

Remind participants that they are now much better informed about falls prevention, and that their answers reflect this.

The Apple Game

Play the Apple Game using questions based on all the major themes (see revision questions at the end of this session outline). Select questions not adequately covered during the above group evaluation. However, time does not always allow for these extra questions.

7.5   GROUP EVALUATION (35 MIN)

Brainstorming activity (again): What causes someone to fall?

Compare this list with the lists saved from Session 1. Note to the group the gains in knowledge about this topic.

This segment (along with an extended break) is the core of today's session. It is very important for the closure of the group and is a powerful reinforcement of many of the major points.

Go around the circle and ask each person:

- What is the major thing you have gained from the program over the last seven weeks?
- Tell the participants you are learning from them and want to improve the next program.

Use that feedback to revise your program and to prepare for the group's three-month follow-up session.

Common statements were:

- 'Well, I'm most grateful. I think I'm walking better. I've been doing the exercises, but I find them quite tiring. My balance has improved, which is the most important one. I actually had a trip last week but I was able to correct myself, which was good because it happened the same way as a fall I've had previously. Scanning ahead is one thing that we've learned that I think is very important.'

- 'I feel I have a better sense of balance; I seem to have more control, particularly on rough footpaths.'

- 'I am more conscious of the spring in my step. I remember the "heel-and-toe"; I am using my feet more.'

- 'I've found the exercises marvellous. I got up every morning to do some of them. I'm starting to find that I'm getting more strength. Also, the safety thing. If you keep your mind aware, then it's good.'

- 'How grateful we are you have put time into helping us older people with our little problems, but getting them as little problems stops them from becoming big problems, we're getting them at the ground roots. I've even dropped my Prednisone by 1 mg. What I like about the groups is that you talk to us not down at us.'

- 'I did have a fall two weeks ago, but it was because I was moving too quickly to get out of a car. Even if the bus is coming, I have learned to slow down. I still tend to rush, but I'm learning.'

- 'You sort of think they are too easy [the exercises]. That's why you do them, because they are easy. They definitely work.'

- 'I found the first few sessions not helpful as I do a lot of exercise. Everyone seemed to be pussyfooting around, but it's been working out. When I got the weights I knew I was on the right track.'

- 'You don't feel like you're on your own. I changed my doctor and have one that listens to me now.'

- 'I am more aware of possible hazards at home. I hold onto something over the shower hob and watch out for the steps and hose.'

- 'Other places never gave us the "why" to do things, and so you stop after several weeks because you don't understand why you need to do things. Even using a bus, I make sure the bus driver knows we have special needs. And I can be assertive, so we manage much better. My balance is better now. When you leave the hospital they say, "You must do this," and don't say what you're getting out of it. We really got something out of this.'

- 'I thought I was observant, but now I'm noticing little things. I'm using the rails on the stairs, which I never used to, because that's what they are there for. I have a neighbour that visits every Wednesday afternoon and says: "Now, what did we learn today?"'

- 'I'm just much more aware of pedestrian crossings and the traffic in general.'
- 'Thank you to the facilitators for their infectious enthusiasm. They have looked on us as people and not as people with grey hair.'

End with: 'Do you think falls can be prevented?'

It is the last session, so make it FUN!

Acknowledge how far they have come, what safety strategies they now have, and how their gains have to be maintained – that exercises are for life.

Talk about what they are going to do after the group finishes.

7.6 FAREWELLS AND FOLLOW-UP (10 MIN)

Give out signed graduation certificates.

Explain that Stepping On has some follow-up activities that participants can expect to hear more about.

A home visit or phone call: This is an opportunity to ask any final questions and to get assistance with adaptations that may need to be made at home. An appointment is scheduled for this meeting.

Booster session(s): Provide the date and an invitation for each participant for the booster session. This session runs for 1.5 hours rather than 2. Past groups have found a get-together in three months to be helpful as a booster and catch-up and this was found to be important in the Stepping On randomised trial.

Are you running more programs? Don't miss this recruitment opportunity but have advertising flyers ready. Ask participants to tell a friend about the Stepping On program.

Thank everyone for being part of the program.

We also send out letters to their GPs –see 'Part 3: Resources'.

The Apple Game quiz: revision

Use this quiz to generate discussion and problem-solving.

Choose what you think is the answer that will best help prevent a fall for you.

What do you do? What could you do?

What might be the barriers?

What would make it easier to follow through and do it?

Community safety:

When I am in a hurry and have to cross a busy street, I:

  (a) cross in the middle of the block so I don't waste time going
      to the light and crossing
  (b) take the extra time to go to the light and cross on a fresh
      green light
  (c) go to the light and cross on the red if there are no cars coming.

Medication management:

Research has proven that taking sedatives does cause falls. So, to help
me get a good night's sleep, instead of taking sedatives, I:

  (a) don't have a bedtime ritual – I do something different each
      night before I go to sleep
  (b) have a clock beside the bed and check the time every time
      I wake up
  (c) go to bed only when I'm ready for sleeping
  (d) am not very active
  (e) drink lots of coffee at night and with dinner.

To prevent falls caused by the kinds of medications I take, I:

  (a) don't want to ask my physician to review my medications
      because he might think I doubt his memory
  (b) never ask my doctor about the side effects of medications.
      He would tell me if I needed to know
  (c) rearrange my schedule so I can take extra care for a couple of
      days when I have new medications that might have unwanted
      side effects
  (d) don't have time to sit and chat with the pharmacist, though my
      neighbour tells me he has found a friendly pharmacist who will
      take the time to tell him about any side effects.

To prevent falls caused by how I take my medications, I:

(a) always take my medications after a meal because that's just what I have always done
(b) never throw any medications out, just in case I might need them
(c) have an infallible memory – I never double up on my medications
(d) always carefully check when, how often, and with what foods I need to take my medications.

Vision and falls:

To make sure my vision doesn't contribute to falls, I:

(a) won't do anything about my cataracts just yet, though I know they're not good
(b) always wear my bifocals or trifocals when walking up or down stairs
(c) have my eyes checked once a year
(d) don't clean my glasses regularly
(e) buy 25-watt bulbs because it saves me money on my power bill.

Footwear:

When I buy new shoes, I:

(a) check the soles to see if they are non-slip
(e) buy the most expensive shoes because they must be safe
(f) buy shoes with leather soles.

When I buy new shoes I think about:

(a) slip, slop and slap
(b) support, fit and sole
(g) good leg to heaven and bad leg to hell.

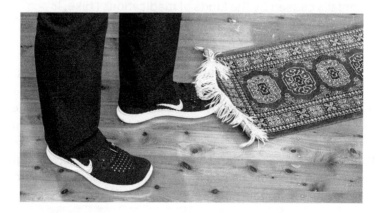

Dizziness

Dizziness is one of the most common symptoms that bring an older person to visit their doctor. Dizziness can increase the risk of falling. 'Dizzy' is a word used to mean a variety of sensations – light-headedness, feeling an abnormal sense of motion, or feeling weak or unsteady.

Dizziness, like balance problems and falling, is too often accepted as a natural part of ageing. Such attitudes do not encourage people to find out what can be done to recover from and to manage dizziness. We have included this information so that the facilitator can be alert to persistent dizziness problems, the types of dizziness problems, the range of management strategies, and when referrals may be required.

Determine what sensations a person is talking about when they say they feel dizzy. It can be difficult to describe, but often can be narrowed down to a few categories:

- light-headedness
- vertigo
- disequilibrium.

Light-headedness

Descriptions of light-headedness may include:

- 'feeling like I will faint'
- head is weightless
- wooziness
- fogginess or cloudiness
- sensation of floating
- giddiness.

Causes of light-headedness:

- decreased blood flow in the brain, caused by:
  - poor response to changing positions against gravity, for example, going from lying to sitting or sitting to standing
  - change in blood pressure with eating, urinating, or bowel movements
  - decreased total blood volume as a result of severe dehydration from vomiting, diarrhoea or fever

- partially blocked arteries (atherosclerosis)
- disease of the heart muscle (cardiomyopathy)
- abnormal heart rhythm (arrhythmia)
- decreased red blood cells carrying oxygen (anaemia)
- low blood sugar
- low carbon dioxide (hyperventilation)
- anxiety
- certain medications. Medications commonly associated with light-headedness include those that affect blood flow or blood sugar.

Common strategies for treating light-headedness:

- sitting on the side of the bed for a few minutes after lying down before getting up
- performing ankle pumps and hand clenching before standing up from sitting, or when standing for a long time
- standing for a few minutes before walking
- encouraging fluid intake if no congestive heart failure (CHF) or other condition that restricts fluid intake
- discussing support stockings with physician
- reviewing medications with physician
- using a cane or walker when standing.

Vertigo

Vertigo is defined as an abnormal sensation of movement of self or surroundings. Descriptions of vertigo may include:

- spinning
- rocking
- waves
- tilting
- prolonged sense of movement after stopping
- may be associated with nausea and vomiting.

Causes of vertigo:

- motion sickness from cars, trains, planes, or amusement rides
- problems with the inner ear (vestibular), caused by:
  - calcium crystals breaking loose (benign paroxysmal positional vertigo)
  - infection or inflammation of the inner ear (acute vestibular neuronitis or labyrinthitis)
  - increased fluid pressure, Meniere's disease
  - antibiotics that damage the ear

- problems with the brain, including:
  - sensory conflict problems
  - migraine
  - stroke
  - vertebrobasilar insufficiency
  - multiple sclerosis
  - tumours, acoustic neuroma or other
  - anxiety.

Common strategies for treating vertigo:

- medication review by a GP
- regular vision check-ups
- treatments for motion sickness approved by a physician. This can include sensory retraining
- consulting an ear, nose and throat (ENT) specialist for inner ear problems
- physical therapy specialising in vestibular rehabilitation for certain inner ear problems and certain central nervous system problems
  - sensory integration training
  - calcium crystal repositioning for BPPV
  - balance training
  - eye coordination training
- using a walking stick, cane or other device for increased sensory input.

Disequilibrium

Someone may use 'dizziness' to describe unsteadiness or imbalance:

- may say 'I felt dizzy on my feet'
- may describe swaying when standing up, but they are not light-headed.

Causes of disequilibrium:

- inner ear (vestibular) problems
- vision abnormalities
- peripheral neuropathy
- joint and muscle problems (muscle weakness and osteoarthritis)
- medications.

Common strategies for treating disequilibrium:

- pain management
- walking stick, cane or other device for increased sensory input with muscle weakness or help with pain management
- balance and strength exercises
- physical therapy for individualised balance and strength training.

Participants who report dizziness should see their doctor to help determine the cause. The timing and triggers of dizziness are often more important than symptom description.

It is helpful to write down:

- a description of the dizziness
- if it occurred suddenly or gradually
- how often it happens
- what makes it worse
- what makes it better.

Tell participants to seek immediate medical advice if they experience any unexplained, recurrent or severe dizziness especially along with any of the following:

- a new, different or severe headache
- blurred vision
- hearing loss
- speech impairment
- leg or arm weakness
- loss of consciousness
- falling or difficulty walking
- numbness or tingling
- chest pain or rapid or slow heart rate.

The follow-up home visit or phone call

OBJECTIVES

1. To assist participants with follow-through of fall prevention strategies and activities
2. To reinforce those fall prevention activities that have been accomplished
3. To support and, if necessary, assist, participants in putting into practice the safety strategies they have been learning within their home and community environments
4. To supplement participant assessments of fall hazards in and about the home
5. To assist with home adaptations and modifications if required
6. To assist with referral to support services upon request.

RESOURCES FOR THE HOME VISIT

Handouts and flyers: local home handyman referrals if available

Other resources: ankle weights for upgrading; commonly used items for sale: walking stick with reflector tape attached or adhesive for mats and other non-slip products.

When a home visit is not possible, consider a follow-up phone call.

FOLLOW-UP

This is a broad-based visit and a time for individual follow-up and positive reinforcement of strategies. Review how they are coping generally. Review how they are managing the exercises: where and when they do them, and how the routine is working for them.

Ask if they are doing anything differently at home or when moving about the community. What changes have been made in and about their home, or again, what things might they be more aware of or do differently? Positively reinforce their decisions and plans. Then assist with plans. They are in control.

BOUNCE BACK IN MY STEP

On a home visit, Nancy told Megan that since the group she had had one fall. She had tripped over a bag when she was tired. She talked about what she had got out of the group. Before the program, she had had quite a few falls outside. She was not enjoying walking, was walking very tensely with her shoulders stooped. She has found now that she scans ahead and does the 'heel-and-toe'. She is much less tense and she is much less stooped. Neighbours have commented that she has her bounce back in her step. She is now enjoying walking. This is a good example of breaking the cycle: getting fitter, feeling confident and feeling in control. She says, 'But we all do it. Now it happens when we're tired and lazy. Most of my problems are when I'm tired and that's when I don't heel-and-toe.'

HOME FALLS HAZARDS

The home visit is an opportunity to support follow-through with hazards that they have identified and to assist with addressing any additional hazards jointly identified during the visit.

Discuss and plan together solutions regarding any hazards in and about the home that have not already been dealt with. Together, check the home for any further hazards, using the Westmead Home Safety Assessment[1] as a guideline (depending on the completeness of the check achieved by the participant). The aim is for the participant to learn to check for hazards and to be aware of the full range of possibilities inside and outside the home, though the occupational therapist may offer expertise and make recommendations.

Identifying home falls hazards has a different focus from the usual occupational therapy home visit, which tends to concentrate on 'ease of doing' and not always on trip or slip hazards along walkways. The Westmead Home Safety Assessment has been designed to identify fall hazards systematically and comprehensively.[2] Its comprehensive nature means that it is a good training tool to alert even experienced therapists to the full range of fall hazards. Therapists may choose to use the Westmead Assessment on occasion to ensure their observation skills are accurate.

---

1   The Westmead Home Safety Assessment can be downloaded from https://fallspreventiononlineworkshops.com.au/.
2   Clemson, Fitzgerald, et al., 1999; Clemson, Fitzgerald, & Heard, 1999.

Simple changes like step edge adhesive strips and reflector tape on canes can be handled on the visit.

Information about local gardening and maintenance services is sometimes useful. This may help with overhanging shrubs or keeping pathways free of moss and leaves. Be aware if someone is still falling. People who fall frequently and recurrently can have, for example, a specific neurological reason and may need a medical referral.

> Remind people to remember to lift their feet up off the ground and walk heel–toe, scanning ahead for hazards.

REFERRALS

Referrals to support services, social supports, and community access: provide assistance with referrals to support services as requested. For example, the person may have thought about a referral to a vision clinic, pharmacist, physical therapist, and so on. Mention My Aged Care registration again.

We found that our program was an opportunity for many people to enhance their social networks. This occurred in the form of ongoing social contact between some group members, and also involved sharing of information by group members in their various other activities and community organisations. Some people may need a little extra direction in connecting with a local organisation.

HOME VISIT OR PHONE CALL?

Some services do not have the capacity to do a follow-up home visit. The US experience has found that a phone call instead of a home visit may be sufficient.

LETTER TO FAMILY DOCTOR

Send a letter to the family doctor, with the person's permission, to advise of the participant's involvement in and outcomes from Stepping On. A suggested template is included below.

Address

Date

Dear Doctor

RE:

Mr/Mrs … recently attended the falls prevention program Stepping On: Building Confidence and Reducing Falls. The aim of the program is to minimise falls risk factors in people over the age of 70. Stepping On is a seven-week community-based program that includes multidisciplinary education about falls prevention in the home and community, and introduces strength and balance training.

Stepping On includes a follow-up home visit with the participant two weeks after the program. This follow-up reinforces newly learned safety strategies and exercises from the program, helps with any referrals that are needed and not yet initiated (such as to an occupational therapist for a home safety assessment), and provides general advice about physical activities available in their local area.

Your patient also has the opportunity to attend a group booster session three months after the program, in which the group will be invited to review their progress, discuss any issues, and revise the exercises and information presented during the program.

Recommendations given to your patient during the program include:

- discussing the risk of medication-related falls and the possibility of a Home Medicines Review with yourself or a pharmacist
- participating in exercises to improve leg strength and balance, and consulting a physiotherapist if experiencing difficulties
- filling out a 'Home safety checklist' and having a home visit from an occupational therapist if needed
- visiting an optometrist for an eye examination

- seeking foot-care services from a podiatrist or foot-care nurse
- having a bone mineral density scan to check for osteoporosis risk.

If you have any questions, please do not hesitate to contact the course facilitator.

Yours sincerely,

Stepping On facilitator's name

Address:

Phone:

Session 8
—
Three-month booster session

OBJECTIVES

The objectives of the three-month follow-up session are:

1. to listen to and acknowledge the ways in which the participants have applied safety strategies in their daily lives since the program
2. to review ways of 'keeping it happening', in particular the exercises
3. to review key points from the program and reinforce skills that the participants have mastered and put into practice
4. to practise the exercises if requested.

RESOURCES FOR SESSION 8

Session materials: Session 8 agenda; name tags; attendance sheet; door signs; display board and display items.

Handouts and flyers: spare 'Balance and strength exercise manual'; Apple Game quiz; community service flyers for exercise groups.

Catering: snacks and beverages for break, apples for Apple Game.

Other resources: leg weights; extension cord.

Outline of Session 8: Booster session: review achievements

8.1 WELCOME 15 MIN	Welcome back. Remind people of housekeeping items. 'In this session we will recap some of the things we've learned from our seven sessions and find out what we're doing now, and how some of us might be keeping these things happening. How did you keep on doing things? What barriers have you faced and how did you overcome these? We can learn from each other in this way. We also want to be sure to review anything you particularly want to go over today.' 'Now, is there anything in particular you would like to revise today? Let us know so that we can be sure to cover it.'
8.2 REVIEW PROGRESS 20 MIN	We're going to start finding out what you have been applying in your everyday lives. What are you doing differently since the last session? The facilitator begins with a personal story; then, if present, a lay leader gives an example of something that changed for them. Each of the participants is then asked to tell of the changes they have put into practice.
8.3 COPING WITH NEGATIVE STORIES AND FALL STORIES 5 MIN	Ask participants to tell their stories and assist them to reframe the events into uselful experiences.
BREAK 15 MIN	

8.4 EXERCISE REVIEW **20 MIN**	This next segment is important as it helps focus on how to keep doing things that are important for preventing falls. 'How do *you* remember to keep doing the exercises? What makes *you* keep doing them? We want you to share this with one another so we can help one another learn.' Choose someone to begin, and ask each person in turn.
8.5 STRENGTH AND BALANCE EXERCISES **10 MIN**	If any exercises were selected by group members, everyone does them together. Discuss the leg weights, and upgrade them where requested.
8.6 BRIEF REVIEW OF KEY ISSUES **20 MIN**	Revision questions for key areas not already raised. The Apple Game. Farewells and refreshments (if available).

8.1 WELCOME (15 MIN)

Welcome back. Remind people of the housekeeping items. 'In this session, we will recap some of the things we've learned from our seven sessions and find out what we're doing now, and how some of us might be keeping these things happening. How did you keep on doing things? What barriers have you faced? And how did you overcome these barriers? We can learn from each other this way. We also want to be sure to review anything you particularly want to go over today.' Review achievements and discuss 'How to keep it going'.

Ask participants: 'Now, is there anything in particular you would like to revise today? Let us know so that we can be sure to cover it.'

8.2 REVIEW PROGRESS (20 MIN)

This segment elicits stories from the participants about safety strategies they are now using or something they have changed or applied in their everyday lives. The facilitator uses a personal short story to get the ball rolling. Then each participant is asked to share something they have changed.

8.3 COPING WITH NEGATIVE STORIES AND FALL STORIES (5 MIN)

Let people tell their stories. If they do not move past the telling and on to evaluating the circumstances and reframing the event into a useful experience, then prompt to help them get there. Assist in reframing to show participants that they can be in control, and remind them that they have new skills in understanding all the things that may have contributed to the situation. What have they done since to prevent falls? They now know things that they can do. Encourage some storytelling.

Keith had recurrent falls before the program. He was not in good health, but had noticed that his strength was much better with the exercises. Shortly after the program, he and his wife moved to a new, small home, leaving behind the family home of 48 years. He had a bad fall on the day of the move at the new front steps and ended up in the hospital. The group talked about the stress and upheaval of moving. Keith remarked how he was now walking a lot more in the new neighbourhood and was back on track with the exercises. He demonstrated a resolve to overcome obstacles along the way. The 'story' only emerged fully because he was prompted to relate the reasons for the fall and the group was prompted to contribute. Then he was prompted to relate what had been happening since the fall and the group was asked to contribute again.

8.4   EXERCISE REVIEW (20 MIN)

Some of the participants will have mentioned exercise in the above segment, but here we want each participant to think about *what keeps them doing the exercises?* or *what barriers have caused them to stop?* We do not expect everyone to be following through, but most people are likely to be doing so at this stage, and they can help boost one another. There is great value in the participants talking about what motivates them, what they get out of doing the exercises, and how these have been incorporated into their daily lives. Other group members can be supported when they are having difficulties. There is opportunity to highlight what has been working for some and also to evaluate the kinds of barriers people have faced. This is also an opportunity to remind participants about exercise groups in the local community.

8.5   STRENGTH AND BALANCE EXERCISES (10 MIN)

Practise the exercises, allowing time for questions and checking on the status of participants using leg weights.

8.6   BRIEF REVIEW OF KEY ISSUES (20 MIN)

Choose questions that will highlight key areas not already raised in the session. This will prompt examples from the group, illustrating what they have put into practice.

For example:

Question: 'Do you remember Katie's talk on vision? A major point raised was to have regular eye checks. Who has regular eye checks? Why is this important for falls prevention?'

Answer: To find out about any deterioration or changes; to check for any disease, e.g. glaucoma (there is a strong link between visual problems and falls); to check for cataracts; having poorer vision in one eye can affect the ability to see edges of steps and other things, and it can affect depth perception.

Questions: 'What do you remember from Shirley's medication talk?'

Answers: To have a physician review of medications; information about unwanted side effects and when to take special care

Question: 'What have people found useful?'

Answers: The 'Personal medication record card'; making a list of questions before the doctor visit; ideas to help sleep instead of taking medications.

Question: 'We talked about lighting at home as being important. Has anyone done anything about that?' Prompt for what has been done and the range of options that could be used.

Questions: 'What about mats around the home? What have you done about these?'

Answers: Removed them, or replaced them with good quality rubber-backed mats, fastened to the floor with the right kind of tape (carpet-to-mat or floor-to-mat tape), or rearranged carpets so they are anchored with furniture, and not in walkways

Question: 'What do the exercises do for you?'

Answers: It helps me not to shuffle, they improve my balance, they improve strength of lower limbs, they give me confidence, they protect me against falls or from injury in falling, they help me keep my independence.

Question: 'How do you find the weights?'

THE APPLE GAME QUIZ, USING GENERAL REVISION QUESTIONS

Allow time for this important part of the session. It may be the last time for participants to support one another and help reinforce their individual achievements. Participants will have let you know the things they have been doing in response to the prompts during the sessions.

Mary revealed she was now walking much more, and feeling more confident and much better. By having a long walk each day (in which she 'heel-and-toes'!), she does not need sleeping tablets. This was reinforced on her vacation, when she had not walked as much and felt like she needed a sleeping tablet. She also made the connection as to why she did not really need a sleeping tablet. This session was an opportunity to validate her achievement, allow her to articulate it and reflect on it, and to help her to keep doing it.

To make the review more interactive, we have at times used two teams and held a competition to see which team remembered the most correct key messages from the seven weeks.

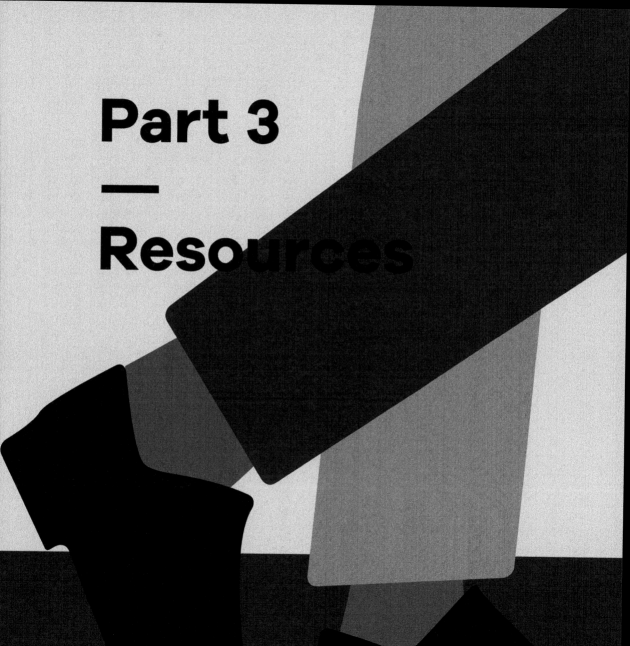

Part 3
—
Resources

Stepping On program facilitator supplies

Name tags:

- Reusable plastic covers with clips

Leg weights:

- Available from various online outlets (www.australian barbell.com.au) plus sports stores such as Rebel and Sportstek. Other cheaper options are available from outlets like Priceline, Big W, Kmart, Aldi.

Strength and balance exercises for participants:

- 'Balance and strength exercise manual', also referred to as the exercise manual and available online. These exercises can be copied for all participants, provided the Stepping On manual has been purchased and copyright is attributed to authors.

For facilitators and physiotherapists:

- The Otago Exercise Program is an example of a relatively intensive home-based exercise program. It is essential background reading for presenting physiotherapists and is also helpful for facilitators. More information available at: The Otago Exercise Program, Carolina Geriatric Education Center, UNC Center for Aging & Health, www.med.unc.edu/aging /cgec/exercise-program
- Fiatarone Singh, M. A. (2000). Chapter 2: The exercise prescription. In M. A. Fiatarone Singh (Ed.), *Exercise, nutrition, and the older woman: wellness for women over fifty* (pp. 38–75 & 93–104). London: CRC Press.

Stepping On handouts and posters:

- These are available online and can be freely copied, provided an acknowledgement is included.

Home safety ladder:

- Lightweight, three- or four-step, fold-up stepladder with safety rail and wide treads.
- These ladders are available from hardware stores.

Stepping On home falls hazards slide presentation:

- Downloadable from the website sydneyuniversitypress.com.au/stepping-on-2019
- Slide version available from Vision Graphics, sales@visiongraphics.com.au, St Leonards NSW, 02 9902 4000

Prince of Wales Medical Research Institute (POWMRI) Quickscreen clinical falls risk assessment screen:

- Falls and Balance Research Group, Prince of Wales Medical Research Institute, Barker Street, Randwick NSW 2031, 02 9399 1005

Continence brochures:

- The Continence Foundation of Australia provides free resources for individuals, carers and professionals to help treat bladder and bowel control problems. Call National Continence Help Line 1800 330 066 or check www.continence.org.au/pages/resources.html.

Public toilet map:

- The Toilet Map (available at www.toiletmap.gov.au) provides information on over 19,000 publicly available toilets across Australia, including accessibility, opening hours and facilities.

Personal alarm systems:

- The following links provide either monitored or unmonitored personal alarms. This information is from the Independent Living Centre Australia and is worth checking updates.
https://ilcaustralia.org.au/search_category_paths/1085
https://ilcaustralia.org.au/search_category_paths/1084
https://ilcaustralia.org.au/search_category_paths/1098

Red Cross Telecross:

- This is a free daily telephone call if you register through MyAgedCare www.redcross.org.au/telecross.aspx

NPS MedicineWise:

Call 1300 134 237; medication lists can be requested and will be mailed to you. The following are now on the NPS website and can be downloaded:

- return your unwanted medicines
- adverse medicine events line (magnet)
- peace of mind with medication
- Medimate
- manage your medicines, manage your health
- Home Medicines Review

MyAgedCare:

- Have brochures on MyAgedCare available because it is the main entry point to the aged care system in Australia. www.myagedcare.gov.au, 1800 200 422
- Emphasise to register for MyAgedCare as it is the portal for many community services.

Stepping On training:

- Within Australia, training is conducted by Megan Swann. For information and enquiries: www.steppingon.com

Bus and train information:

- A link to all Australian bus transport websites: www.busaustralia.com

Information on timetables with special assistance for each state

ACT	13 17 10
	www.transport.act.gov.au
	www.transport.act.gov.au/about-us /accessible-travel
NORTHERN TERRITORY	https://nt.gov.au/driving
NSW	13 15 00
	https://transportnsw.info
	https://transportnsw.info/travel-info /using-public-transport/accessible-travel
QUEENSLAND	13 12 30
	www.translink.com.au
	https://translink.com.au/travel-with-us /accessibility
SOUTH AUSTRALIA	1300 311 108
	www.adelaidemetro.com.au
	www.adelaidemetro.com.au /Using-Adelaide-Metro/Accessibility-Disability
TASMANIA	https://www.transport.tas.gov.au
VICTORIA	1800 800 007
	www.metlinkmelbourne.com.au
	www.ptv.vic.gov.au/more /travelling-on-the-network/accessibility
WESTERN AUSTRALIA	13 62 13
	www.transperth.wa.gov.au
	www.transperth.wa.gov.au /Using-Transperth/Station-Facilities

Guide dogs, orientation and mobility:

- Guide Dogs NSW/ACT: www.guidedogs.com.au, 02 9412 9300
- Macular Disease Foundation Australia: www.mdfoundation.com.au, 1800 111 709

Vision Australia:

- www.visionaustralia.org.au, 1800 331 000

Osteoporosis Australia:

- www.osteoporosis.org.au, 1800 242 141
- Articles on the importance of calcium, vitamin D and exercise for osteoporosis prevention are available on www.osteoporosis.org.au/prevention
- 'What you need to know about osteoporosis: consumer guide', 4th edition, 2016/17, https://bit.ly/2n5f2u5

Culturally and linguistically diverse (CALD) resources

Exercises:

- Australian Physiotherapy Association: www.physiotherapy.asn.au, 02 8748 1555

Home safety hazards:

- Occupational Therapy Association of Australia: www.otaus.com.au, 02 9648 3225

Calcium and vitamin D:

- Dietitians Association of Australia: www.daa.asn.au, 1800 812 942

Pedestrian safety:

- The Multicultural Community Liaison Officer (MCLO) program employs civilian officers at the local level to work with communities and police to strengthen links and facilitate communication and interaction between police and culturally and linguistically diverse (CALD) communities. MCLOs identify local priorities for police and culturally diverse communities, encourage partnerships, and forge better relationships between police officers and members of the community. You can speak to an MCLO if you need help to report a crime to police, or to raise any issues of concern with police. MCLOs are located at the following Local Area Commands: Ashfield, Bankstown, Blacktown, Burwood, Cabramatta, Campbelltown, Campsie, City Central (Darling Harbour), Eastwood, Fairfield, Flemington (Auburn), Green Valley, Hurstville, Kuring-gai (Hornsby), Liverpool Holroyd (Merrylands), Macquarie Fields, Manly, Marrickville, Mt Druitt, Northern Beaches (Dee Why), North Shore (Chatswood), Parramatta, Rosehill (Granville), St George (Kogarah) and Wollongong.

- Multicultural Council Worker: contact your local council.
- Australian Driver Training Association: www.adta.com.au, 02 9647 2711

Vision:

- For Guide Dogs NSW/ACT (or check with your local state): www.guidedogs.com.au, 02 9412 9300
- Vision Australia: www.visionaustralia.org, 1300 847 466
- Optometrists Association Australia NSW/ACT Division: www.optometry.org.au/nsw, 02 9712 2199

Pharmaceuticals:

- NPS – MedicineWise: www.nps.org.au, 02 8217 8700

Safe footwear:

- Australian Podiatry Association – NSW & ACT: www.podiatry.asn.au, 02 9698 3751

Triple zero:

- When you ring 000 for an emergency, state your language immediately after they answer, e.g. 'Mandarin Chinese'.

Stepping On resources:

- Sydney University Press has CALD resources online: sydneyuniversitypress.com.au/stepping-on-2019

The display

The display table is set up for each session and is limited to small items that can be easily transported. The following examples are falls-related display items that can be included.

Lighting:

- LED night-light (plugs into power point and gives a constant dim light)
- bedside touch lamp (from hardware, homeware and lighting shops; cheaper brands available)
- fluorescent energy-saving lamps (from hardware and lighting shops)
- light bulb grabber, e.g. HPM globe grabber (assists in replacing light globes in the ceiling)

Slippery surfaces (listed items available from most hardware stores):

- mats for slippery tiles
- anti-moss product
- CPC slip grip for slippery tiles
- bathtub strips
- 3M safety-walk 50 mm × 4.5 m slip-resistant indoor/outdoor black tread (self-adhesive strips for step edges)
- 3M safety-walk step and ladder tread outdoor tread (25 mm × 4.5 m black or 50 mm × 4.5 m black; self-adhesive strips for external steps)

Flooring and mats:

- carpet tape (from hardware stores)
- Velcro carpet-to-carpet tape (from hardware stores)
- rubber latex matting (from Target, Ikea and other homeware stores, and from catalogues)

Security:

- Scotch reflective tape (can be put on bag, raincoat or walking stick; from hardware shops)

- reflective fluoro-tape arm bands (from bicycle shops)
- 3-in-1 soft light (polar pulse light; emergency small lights for handbags or keys)
- information on a credit card security alert system, e.g. Sentinel 02 9937 7350
- key alert (personal handbag alarm)

Mobility aid safety:

- rubber ferrules (rubber stoppers for walking sticks; assorted sizes available)
- walking stick frogs (to hold cane against a table; available from pharmacies)
- examples of fold-down walking sticks (available from chemists)

Telephone:

- cordless telephone

Shoes (from hardware and shoe repair shops):

- rubber soling compound
- shoe treads
- a home repair kit for soles
- shoe repair kit (rubber and adhesive to repair holes in soles)
- elastic shoelaces and shoe horn

Medication management:

- pill master cup and container (also cuts and grinds tablets)
- pill boxes

Local community resources:

- Aged Care Assessment Team information
- Commonwealth Home Support Programme (CHSP) through MyAgedCare
- local council handyman service
- home maintenance and modification service
- Tai Chi and other local physical activity groups that offer standing exercise classes
- Senior Centres and services for older people
- local council activity centres and services for older people
- health promotion leaflets

Medicine record cards:

- Combined Pensioners and Superannuants Association of NSW
- National Prescribing Service (NPS)
- Medi-List (from the Australian government Department of Health Pharmaceutical Benefits Scheme [PBS]) and Health Care Card (from the Australian government Department of Human Services)

Hip protectors:

- www.sanicare.com
- www.hipsaver.com.au

Independent Living Centre:

- For information on other products, contact the Independent Living Centre or LifeTec in your state.

Reference book for Stepping On participants to borrow or purchase:

- *Staying power: tips and tools to keep you on your feet* by Lindy Clemson and Megan Swann. Available from Sydney University Press (sydneyuniversitypress.com.au/staying-power). Email sup.info@sydney.edu.au or phone 02 9036 9958.

Stepping On display items

Below is a list of items that would make a good start for your display table. Introduce new items weekly within your discussion. Find where you can purchase these locally. Some items you may like to purchase and distribute as gifts to participants in Session 7.

SESSION	ITEM	WHERE FROM?	APPROX. PRICE
2	Foldable walking stick	Chemist	$30
2	Walking stick frog/ holder	Medical supplier/ chemist	$6
2	Walking stick rubber ferrules	Chemist/medical supplier	Variable
3	Non-slip strips for bath (often animal print)	Hardware shop	$10
3	Anti-slip contrast tape (range of colours available)	Hardware shop	$7.50
3	Anti-moss and mould product	Hardware shop	$30
3	Carpet tape stick– double sided or Velcro	Hardware shop	From $6

SESSION	ITEM	WHERE FROM?	APPROX. PRICE
3	Bath mats	Homeware shop, department stores.	$10
		The best idea is to explore your local shops, put mats down on the floor and test whether they slip or not.	
3	Non-slip matting	Hardware shop	$5.50/m
4	Personal key-chain alarm	Electrical stores	$10
5	Key-chain torch	Reject Shop, etc.	From $2
5	Narrower reflective tape	Hardware shop	$14
5	Wider reflective tape (could be used on walking aid, scooter, etc. to increase visibility)	Hardware shop	$12
5	LED night-light, auto turn-on in low light	Hardware shop	$10

SESSION	ITEM	WHERE FROM?	APPROX. PRICE
5	Touch lamp	Hardware/ homeware shop	From $20
5	Reflective leg/arm band, vests, stickers	Bicycle shop	$10
6	Long-handled shoehorn (a good gift to give participants)	Chemist, medical supplier or Ikea if you can get there – they limit purchases to 20 per customer, but stock up if you can. These are great!	From $2
6	Pill splitter	Chemist	$10
6	Pill box	Chemist	From $6
6	Webster Pack	Chemist	Ask your local chemist for a free sample pack

Expert speakers

Week 1:

- Physiotherapist (e.g. physical therapist trained in aged care, exercise physiologist, fitness instructor)

Week 2:

- Physiotherapist (e.g. physical therapist trained in aged care, exercise physiologist, fitness instructor)

Week 3:

- Occupational therapist

Week 4:

- Community safety expert (e.g. local council road safety officer)
- Footwear expert (e.g. podiatrist, shoe specialist, occupational therapist, certified pedorthist)

Week 5:

- Vision expert (e.g. Guide Dogs Australia or Vision Australia representative, optometrist, opthamologist)
- Calcium and vitamin D (e.g. dietician, bone health nurse, Osteoarthritis Australia representative)
- Past Stepping On graduate

Week 6:

- Physiotherapist (e.g. physical therapist trained in aged care, exercise physiologist, fitness instructor)
- Medication management expert (e.g. pharmacist)

Week 7:

- Facilitator only

Personal alarm systems

MONITORED

- Baptist Care – Carecall: www.Baptistcare.org.au/carecall, 1300 130 100
- CareAlert: www.carealert.com.au, 1300 758 595
- Constant Companion: 9777 7836, email: constantcompanion@willoughby.nsw.gov.au
- First Call: www.firstcallmedicalalarms.com.au, 1300 408 080
- Safety Link – personal response service: 1800 813 617
- Silent Sentinel – automatic fall detection: www.silentsentinel.com.au, 1300 300 247
- SureSafe: www.personalalarms.net.au, 1300 739 991
- Vital Call: www.vitalcall.com.au, 1300 360 808 or request a free in-home demonstration to get started.

NON-MONITORED

- Livelife personal alarms: livelifealarms.com.au, 03 5744 3580
- Medialarm: www.medialarm.com.au, 1300 665 322
- Mobile alert: www.mobile-alert.com.au, 9705 1888 or 0416 161 073
- Watch alert for android phones: www.rightminder.com

Health organisations

- Healthdirect Australia is a free 24-hour telephone service staffed by registered nurses to provide expert healthy advice: www.healthdirect.org.au, 1800 022 222
- Arthritis & Osteoporosis New South Wales: www.arthritisnsw. org.au, 1800 011 041 (free call in NSW)
- Occupational Therapy Australia: www.otaus.com.au, 02 9648 3225
- Australian Association of Social Workers: www.aasw.asn.au, 02 9518 4944
- Australian Physiotherapy Association: www.physiotherapy. asn.au, 02 8744 1555
- Australian Podiatry Association: www.apodc.com.au, 03 9416 3111
- NSW Falls Prevention Network: fallsnetwork.neura.edu.au
- Active and Healthy: www.activeandhealthy.nsw.gov.au

Stepping On training for facilitators

- In Australia, training for Stepping On facilitators is conducted by Megan Swann. For information and enquiries: www.steppingon.com
- In the USA, training for Stepping On facilitators and 'Train the Trainer' programs are offered by the Wisconsin Institute for Healthy Aging: wihealthyaging.org/stepping-on

ONLINE HOME SAFETY LEARNING MODULE:

- www.fallspreventiononlineworkshops.com.au/ see under Allied Health: Home & Community Online module
- Online training for occupational therapists in conducting home safety home visits
- The Falls Prevention Home and Community Safety Online Workshop is designed to train occupational therapists and other health-care providers in how to conduct a comprehensive home visit (with evidence-based best practice) to reduce the risk of falls for older community-residing adults. It aims to train the therapist to work together with the older person: to identify environmental hazards and behavioural risks, to raise awareness of risks, and to jointly find solutions.
- Presented in six modules, this workshop provides the tools for and the clinical reasoning underpinning the intervention, and includes case studies illustrating applications of the approach.

Other books

Available from Sydney University Press, Amazon.com and Book Depository:

STAYING POWER: TIPS AND TOOLS TO KEEP YOU ON YOUR FEET

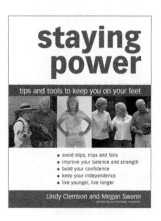

Lindy Clemson and Megan Swann-Williams

The key to healthy ageing is to adopt a positive, confident attitude and to stay connected to your community. *Staying power: tips and tools to keep you on your feet* gives practical and inspirational advice on how to prevent falls in your life. Through a combination of exercise and a healthy, active approach, you can beat what seem like the inevitable outcomes of getting older.

The ideas in *Staying power* are based on Stepping On program, which has successfully changed the lives of many older people. That program has reduced the fall rate of its participants by over 30 per cent. The book is packed with ideas for setting up your home, getting out and about in your community, and developing balance and strength in your body, as well as success stories from older people who have adopted these habits. *Staying power* will have you on your feet in no time and will keep you there.

LIFESTYLE-INTEGRATED FUNCTIONAL EXERCISE (LiFE) PROGRAM TO PREVENT FALLS

Lindy Clemson, Jo Munro and Maria Fiatarone Singh

LiFE is an individual program of activities embedded into daily routines and tasks. In a randomised control trial published in the *British Medical Journal* in 2012, the risk of falls in older people was reduced by one-third, the ability to do everyday tasks was improved, and physical activity levels increased. LiFE is a different approach to a traditional exercise program. In the LiFE program, unloading the dishwasher can become an opportunity to improve strength. Brushing your teeth can become a chance to improve balance. Your home or your garden can be your 'gym'. LiFE activities are tailored to individual lifestyles. The LiFE manuals will introduce you to the key elements of LiFE, the underpinning concepts, and embedding LiFE activities into your daily routines and strategies in order to habits.

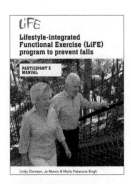

PARTICIPANT'S MANUAL

The *Participant's manual* provides detailed descriptions of the strength and balance activities and outlines the principles of LiFE. It shows how the activities can be incorporated into an everyday routine and includes several stories of successful participants.

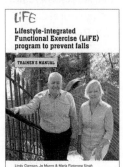

TRAINER'S MANUAL

The *Trainer's manual* presents the conceptual underpinning of the LiFE program and provides a step-by-step guide for therapists and trainers to implement LiFE with their clients.

Works cited

Adelman, R. D., Greene, M. G., & Ory, M. G. (2000). Communication between older patients and their physicians. *Clinics in Geriatric Medicine, 16*(1), 1–25.

Ades, P. A., Ballor, D. L., Ashikaga, T., Utton, J. L., & Nair, K. S. (1996). Weight training improves walking endurance in healthy elderly persons. *Annals of Internal Medicine, 124*(6), 568–572. doi: 10.7326/0003-4819-124-6-199603150-00005

American College of Sports Medicine, Chodzko-Zajko, W. J., Proctor, D. N., Fiatarone Singh, M. A., Minson, C. T., Nigg, C. R., ... Skinner, J. S. (2009). American College of Sports Medicine position stand. Exercise and physical activity for older adults. *Medicine & Science in Sports & Exercise, 41*(7), 1510–1530. doi: 10.1249/MSS.0b013e3181a0c95c

Bales, R. F. (1950). *Interaction process analysis.* Cambridge, MA: Addison Wesley.

Bandura, A. (1977). Self-efficacy: toward a unifying theory of behavioural change. *Psychological Review, 84*, 191–215. doi: 10.1037/0033-295X.84.2.191

Bandura, A. (1986). *Social foundations of thought and action: a social cognitive theory.* Englewood Cliffs, NJ: Prentice-Hall.

Bandura, A. (1995). *Self-efficacy in a changing society.* Cambridge, UK: Cambridge University Press.

Bandura, A. (1997). *Self-efficacy: the exercise of control.* New York, NY: W. H. Freeman.

Bath, P. A., & Morgan, K. (1999). Differential risk factor profiles for indoor and outdoor falls in older people living at home in Nottingham, UK. *European Journal of Epidemiology, 15*(1), 65–73. doi: 10.1023/A:1007531101765

Black, D. S., O'Reilly, G. A., Olmstead, R., Breen, E. C., & Irwin, M. R. (2015). Mindfulness meditation and improvement in sleep quality and daytime impairment among older adults with sleep disturbances: a randomized clinical trial. *JAMA Internal Medicine, 175*(4), 494–501. doi: 10.1001/jamainternmed.2014.8081

Bleijlevens, M. H. C., Diederiks, J. P. M., Hendriks, M. R. C., van Haastregt, J. C. M., Crebolder, H., & van Eijk, J. T. M. (2010). Relationship between location and activity in injurious falls: an exploratory study. *BMC Geriatrics, 10*(1), 40. doi: 10.1186/1471-2318-10-40

Boud, D., Keogh, R., & Walker, D. (1985). Chapter 1. Promoting reflection in learning: a model. In D. Boud (Ed.), *Reflection: turning experience into learning* (pp. 18–40). New York, NY: Nichols.

Bradley, C., & Pointer, S. (2008). Hospitalisations due to falls by older people, Australia 2005–06. *Injury Research and Statistics Series, 50*, 1444–3791.

Brookfield, S. D., & Preskill, S. (1999). *Discussion as a way of teaching.* Buckingham, UK: The Society for Research into Higher Education & Open University Press.

Campbell, A. J., Reinken, J., Allan, B. C., & Martinez, G. S. (1981). Falls in old age: a study of frequency and related clinical factors. *Age and Ageing, 10*(4), 264–270. doi: 10.1093/ageing/10.4.264

Campbell, A. J., Robertson, M. C., Gardner, M. M., Norton, R., & Buchner, D. M. (1999). Psychotropic medication withdrawal and a home-based exercise program to prevent falls: a randomized, controlled trial. *Journal of the American Geriatrics Society, 47*(7), 850–853. doi: 10.1111/j.1532-5415.1999.tb03843.x

Campbell, A. J., Robertson, M. C., Gardner, M. M., Norton, R. N., Tilyard, M. W., & Buchner, D. M. (1997). Randomised controlled trial of a general practice programme of home based exercise to prevent falls in elderly women. *British Medical Journal, 315*(7115), 1065–1069. doi: 10.1136/bmj.315.7115.1065

Campbell, A. J., Robertson, M. C., La Grow, S. J., Kerse, N. M., Sanderson, G. F., Jacobs, R. J., … Hale, L. A. (2005). Randomised controlled trial of prevention of falls in people aged ≥75 with severe visual impairment: the VIP trial. *British Medical Journal, 331*(7520), 817–820. doi: 10.1136/bmj.38601.447731.55

Carande-Kulis, V., Stevens, J. A., Florence, C. S., Beattie, B. L., & Arias, I. (2015). A cost–benefit analysis of three older adult fall prevention interventions. *Journal of Safety Research, 52*, 65–70. doi: 10.1016/j.jsr.2014.12.007

Carroll, C., Patterson, M., Wood, S., Booth, A., Rick, J., & Balain, S. (2007). A conceptual framework for implementation fidelity. *Implementation Science, 2*(1), 40–49. doi: 10.1186/1748-5908-2-40

Chalk, R. (2000). Working with groups. In A. Compton & M. Ashwin (Eds.), *Community care for health professionals* (2nd edn) (pp. 145–48). Oxford, UK: Butterworth-Heinemann.

Chapuy, M. C., Arlot, M., Duboeuf, F., Brun, J., Coruzet, B., Arnaud, S., … Meunier, P. J. (1992). Vitamin D3 and calcium to prevent hip fractures in elderly women. *New England Journal of Medicine, 327*(23), 1637–1642.

Cheal, B., & Clemson, L. (2001). Older people enhancing self-efficacy in fall risk situations. *Australian Occupational Therapy Journal, 48*(2), 80–91. doi: 10.1046/j.1440-1630.2001.00250.x

Cistulli, P. A., & Singh, N. A. (2000). Sleep. In M. A. Fiatarone Singh (Ed.), *Exercise, nutrition, and the older woman: wellness for women over fifty* (pp. 417–441). London, UK: CRC Press.

Clemson, L. *Home and community safety fall prevention (online module) and Westmead Home Safety Assessment 2016*. Retrieved from www.fallspreventiononlineworkshops.com.au

Clemson, L. (1997). *Home fall hazards and the Westmead Home Safety Assessment*. West Brunswick, Victoria: Co-ordinates Publications. Now updated (2016) as 'Falls Prevention Workshops' www.fallspreventiononlineworkshops.com.au

Clemson, L., Bundy, A., Cumming, R. G., Kay, L. G., & Luckett, T. (2008). Validating the Falls Behavioural (FaB) scale for older people: a Rasch analysis. *Disability and Rehabilitation, 30*(7), 498–506. doi: 10.1080/09638280701355546

Clemson, L., Cumming, R. G., & Heard, R. (2003). The development of an assessment to evaluate behavioural factors associated with falling. *American Journal of Occupational Therapy, 57*(4), 380–388. doi: 10.5014/ajot.57.4.380

Clemson, L., Cumming, R. G., Kendig, H., Swann, M., Heard, R., & Taylor, K. (2004). The effectiveness of a community-based program for reducing the incidence of falls in the elderly: a randomized trial. *Journal of the American Geriatrics Society, 52*(9), 1487–1494. doi: 10.1111/j.1532-5415.2004.52411.x

Clemson, L., Cusick, A., & Fozzard, C. (1999). Managing risk and exerting control: determining follow through with falls prevention. *Disability and Rehabilitation, 21*(12), 531–541. doi: 10.1080/096382899297189

Clemson, L., Cusick, A., & Fozzard, C. (1998). Reducing falls at home: understanding the client's decision-making process. Paper presented at the 12th International Congress of the World Federation of Occupational Therapists, Montreal, QC, May–June 1998.

Clemson, L., Fiatarone Singh, M. A., Bundy, A., Cumming, R. G., Manollaras, K., O'Loughlin, P., & Black, D. (2012). Integration of balance and strength training into daily life activity to reduce rate of falls in older people (the LiFE study): randomised parallel trial. *British Medical Journal, 345*(7870), 14–14. doi: 10.1136/bmj.e4547

Clemson, L., Fitzgerald, M. H., & Heard, R. (1999). Content validity of an assessment tool to identify home fall hazards: the Westmead Home Safety Assessment. *British Journal of Occupational Therapy, 62*(4), 171–179. doi: 10.1177/030802269906200407

Clemson, L., Fitzgerald, M. H., Heard, R., & Cumming, R. G. (1999). Inter-rater reliability of a home fall hazards assessment tool. *Occupational Therapy Journal of Research, 19*(2), 83–98. doi: 10.1177/153944929901900201

Clemson, L., & Munro, J. (2016). Conceptual model of habit reforming to improve balance and prevent falls. In N. A. Pachana (Ed.), *Encyclopaedia of geropsychology* 1st edn: (pp. 1–10). Singapore: Springer.

Clemson, L., Taylor, K., Cumming, R. G., Kendig, H., & Swann, M. (2007). Recruiting older participants to a randomized trial of a community-based falls prevention program. *Australasian Journal of Ageing, 26*(1), 35–39. doi: 10.1111/j.1741-6612.2007.00203.x

Clemson, L., & Swann-Williams, M. (2010). *Staying power: tips and tools to keep you on your feet*. Sydney: Sydney University Press.

Cole, H., Berger, P., & Garrity, T. (1988). Analogues between medical and industrial safety research on compliance behavior. In D. Gochman (Ed.), *Health behaviour: emerging research perspectives* (pp. 337–353). New York, NY: Plenum Press.

Coleman, A. L., Cummings, S. R., Yu, F., Kodjebacheva, G., Ensrud, K. E., Gutierrez, P., … Study Group of Osteoporotic Fractures. (2007). Binocular visual-field loss increases the risk of future falls in older white women. *Journal of the American Geriatrics Society, 55*(3), 357–364. doi:10.1111/j.1532-5415.2007.01094.x

Coleman, P. G. (1999). Identity management in later life. In R. T. Woods (Ed.), *Psychological problems of ageing: assessment, treatment and care* (pp. 49–72). Chichester, UK: John Wiley & Sons.

Cullinan, T. R., Silver, J. H., Gould, E. S., & Irvine, D. (1979). Visual disability and home lighting. *The Lancet, 313*(8117), 642–644. doi:10.1016/S0140-6736(79)91082-1

Cumming, R. G., Ivers, R., Clemson, L., Cullen, J., Hayes, M. F., Tanzer, M., & Mitchell, P. (2007). Improving vision to prevent falls in frail older people: a randomized trial. *Journal of the American Geriatrics Society, 55*(2), 175–181. doi: 10.1111/j.1532-5415.2007.01046.x

Cumming, R. G., Thomas, M., Szonyi, G., Frampton, G., Salkeld, G., & Clemson, L. (2001). Adherence to occupational therapist recommendations for home modifications for falls prevention. *American Journal of Occupational Therapy, 55*(6), 641–648. doi:10.5014/ajot.55.6.641

Cumming, R. G., Thomas, M., Szonyi, G., Salkeld, G., O'Neill, E., Westbury, C., & Frampton, G. (1999). Home visits by an occupational therapist for assessment and modification of environmental hazards: a randomized trial of falls prevention. *Journal of the American Geriatrics Society, 47*(12), 1397–1402. doi: 10.1111/j.1532-5415.1999.tb01556.x

Daly, R. M. (2017). Exercise and nutritional approaches to prevent frail bones, falls and fractures: an update. *Climacteric, 20*(2), 119–124. doi: 10.1080/13697137.2017.1286890

Day, L., Fildes, B., Gordon, I., Fitzharris, M., Flamer, H., & Lord, S. (2002). Randomised factorial trial of falls prevention among older people living in their own homes. *British Medical Journal, 325*(7356), 128–131. doi: 10.1136/bmj.325.7356.128

Day, L., Kent, S., & Fildes, B. (1994). Injuries among older people. In Victorian Injury Surveillance Unit (Ed.), *Hazard, 18*, (pp. 1–16). Melbourne, Victoria: Monash University Accident Research Centre.

de Groot, G., & Fagerström, L. (2011). Older adults' motivating factors and barriers to exercise to prevent falls. *Scandinavian Journal of Occupational Therapy, 18*(2), 153–160. doi:10.3109/11038128.2010.487113

Delbaere, K., Smith, S. T., & Lord, S. R. (2011). Development and initial validation of the Iconographical Falls Efficacy Scale. *Journals of Gerontology Series A – Biological Sciences & Medical Sciences, 66*(6), 674–680. doi:10.1093/gerona/glr019

Denzin, N. K. (1994). The art and politics of interpretation. In N. K. Denzin & Y. S. Lincoln (Eds.), *Handbook of qualitative research* (pp. 500–515). Thousand Oaks, CA: Sage.

Duckham, R. L., Procter-Gray, E., Hannan, M. T., Leveille, S. G., Lipsitz, L. A., & Li, W. J. (2013). Sex differences in circumstances and consequences of outdoor and indoor falls in older adults in the MOBILIZE Boston cohort study. *BMC Geriatrics, 13*(1), 133. doi:10.1186/1471-2318-13-133

Duque, G., Daly, R. M., Sanders, K., & Kiel, D. P. (2017). Vitamin D, bones and muscle: myth versus reality. *Australasian Journal on Ageing, 36*, 8–13. doi: 10.1111/ajag.12407

Egger, G., Spark, R., & Lawson, J. (1990). *Health promotion strategies and methods*. Sydney, NSW: McGraw-Hill Books.

Fiatarone, M. A., Marks, E. C., Ryan, N. D., Meredith, C. N., Lipsitz, L. A., & Evans, W. J. (1990). High-intensity strength training in nonagenarians: effects on skeletal muscle. *Journal American Medical Association, 263*(22), 3029–3034. doi: 10.1001/jama.1990.03440220053029

Fiatarone Singh, M. A. (2000). *Exercise, nutrition, and the older woman: wellness for women over fifty*. London, UK: CRC Press.

Finlay, O. E. (1986). Footwear management in the elderly care programme. *Physiotherapy, 72*(4), 172–178.

Fischoff, B. (1989). Risk: a guide to controversy. In National Research Council (Ed.), *Improving risk communication* (pp. 211–319). Washington, DC: National Academic Press.

Fitzgerald, M. H. (2001). Gaining knowledge of culture during professional education. In J. Higgs & A. Tichen (Eds.), *Practice knowledge and expertise in the health professions* (pp. 149–156). Melbourne, Victoria: Butterworth Heinemann.

Franco, M. R., Tong, A., Howard, K., Sherrington, C., Ferreira, P. H., Pinto, R. Z., & Ferreira, M. L. (2015). Older people's perspectives on participation in physical activity: a systematic review and thematic synthesis of qualitative literature. *British Journal of Sports Medicine, 49*(19), 1268–1276. doi: 10.1136/bjsports-2014-094015

Gage, M., Cook, J. V., & Fryday-Field, K. (1997). Understanding the transition to community living after discharge from an acute care hospital: an exploratory study. *American Journal of Occupational Therapy, 51*(2), 96–103. doi: 10.5014/ajot.51.2.96

Garrett, S. K. M., Thomas, A. P., Cicuttini, F., Silagy, C., Taylor, H. R., & McNeil, J. J. (2000). Community-based recruitment strategies for a longitudinal interventional study: the VECAT experience. *Journal of Clinical Epidemiology, 53*(5), 541–548. doi: 10.1016/S0895-4356(99)00153-5

Geertz, C. (1988). Thick description: toward an interpretive theory of culture. In R. E. Emerson (Ed.), *Contemporary field research: a collection of readings* (pp. 37–59). Prospect Heights, Ill: Waveland Press.

Gillespie, L. D., Robertson, M. C., Robertson, M. C., Gillespie, W. J., Sherrington, C., Gates, S., … Lamb, S. E. (2012). Interventions for preventing falls in older people living in the community. *Cochrane Database of Systematic Reviews (Online), 9*(9), CD007146. doi: 10.1002/14651858.CD007146.pub3

Gitlin, L. (2009). Environmental adaptations for older adults and their families in the home and community. In I. Soderback (Ed.), *International handbook of occupational therapy interventions* (pp. 53–62). London, UK: Springer.

Haines, T., Hill, K., Vu, T., Clemson, L., Finch, C., & Day, L. (2016). Does action follow intention with participation in home and group-based falls prevention exercise programs? An exploratory, prospective, observational study. *Archives of Gerontology & Geriatrics, 64,* 151–161. doi: 10.1016/j.archger.2016.02.003

Haran, M. J., Cameron, I. D., Ivers, R. Q., Simpson, J. M., Lee, B. B., Tanzer, M., ... Lord, S. R. (2010). Effect on falls of providing single lens distance vision glasses to multifocal glasses wearers: VISIBLE randomised controlled trial. *British Medical Journal, 340*(7760), 1345–1345. doi: 10.1136/bmj.c2265

Hare, A., Borgatta, E. F., & Bales, R. F. (1965). *Small groups: studies in social interaction.* New York, NY: Alfred A. Knopf.

Hartley, J. (1998). *Learning and studying: a research perspective.* New York, NY: Routledge.

Harwood, R. H., Foss, A. J., Osborn, F., Gregson, R. M., Zaman, A., & Masud, T. (2005). Falls and health status in elderly women following first eye cataract surgery: a randomised controlled trial. *British Journal of Ophthalmology, 89*(1), 53–59. doi: 10.1136/bjo.2004.049478

Hatton, A. L., Sturnieks, D. L., Lord, S. R., Lo, J. C. M., Menz, H. B., & Menant, J. C. (2013). Effects of nonslip socks on the gait patterns of older people when walking on a slippery surface. *Journal of the American Podiatric Medical Association, 103*(6), 471–479.

Hill, K., Clemson, L., & Vrantsidis, F. (2006). Preventing falls – a key to maintaining independence. In H. Mackey & S. Nancarrow (Eds.), *Enabling independence: a guide for rehabilitation workers* (pp. 182–202). London, UK: Blackwell.

Hill, K. D., Schwartz, J. A., Kalogeropoulos, A. J., & Gibson, S. J. (1996). Fear of falling revisited. *Archives of Physical Medicine & Rehabilitation, 77*(10), 1025–1029. doi: 10.1016/S0003-9993(96)90063-5

Hillsdon, M., Thorogood, M., Anstiss, T., & Morris, J. (1995). Randomised controlled trials of physical activity promotion in free living populations: a review. *Journal of Epidemiology & Community Health, 49*(5), 448–453. doi: 10.1136/jech.49.5.448

Hoch, C. C., Reynolds, C. F., Buysse, D. J., Monk, T. H., Nowell, P., Begley, A. E., ... Dew, M. A. (2001). Protecting sleep quality in later life: a pilot study of bed restriction and sleep hygiene. *Journals of Gerontology – Series B Psychological Sciences and Social Sciences, 56*(1), P52–P59. doi:10.1093/geronb/56.1.P52

Hoyt, M. F., & Janis, I. L. (1982). Increasing adherence to a stressful decision via the Balance-Sheet Procedure: a field experiment on attendance at an exercise class. In I. L. Janis (Ed.), *Counseling on personal decisions: theory and research on short-term helping relationships.* New Haven, CT: Yale University Press.

Huang, Z-G., Feng, Y., Li, Y-H., & Lv, C-S. (2017). Systematic review and meta-analysis: Tai Chi for preventing falls in older adults. *BMJ Open, 7*(2), e013661. doi: 10.1136/bmjopen-2016013661

Ivers, R. Q., Cumming, R. G., Mitchell, P., & Attebo, K. (1998). Visual impairment and falls in older adults: the Blue Mountains Eye Study. *Journal of the American Geriatrics Society, 46*(1), 58–64. doi: 10.1111/j.1532-5415.1998.tb01014.x

Ivers, R. Q., Norton, R., Cumming, R. G., Butler, M., & Campbell, A. J. (2000). Visual impairment and risk of hip fracture. *American Journal of Epidemiology, 152*(7), 633–639. doi: 10.1093/aje/152.7.633

Jang, H., Clemson, L., Lovarini, M., Willis, K., Lord, S. R., & Sherrington, C. (2015). Cultural influences on exercise participation and fall prevention: a systematic review and narrative synthesis. *Disability and Rehabilitation,* 1–9. doi: 10.3109/09638288.2015.1061606

Janis, I. L., & Mann, L. (1977). *Decision-making: a psychological analysis of conflict, choice, and commitment.* New York, NY: Macmillan Publishing.

Jacques, D. (1991). *Learning in groups.* London, UK: Kogan Page.

Jacques, D., & Salmon, G. (2008). *Learning in groups: a handbook for face-to-face and online environments* (4th edn). New York, NY: Routledge.

Kelsey, J. L., Procter-Gray, E., Hannan, M. T., & Li, W. J. (2012). Heterogeneity of falls among older adults: implications for public health prevention. *American Journal of Public Health, 102*(11), 2149–2156. doi: 10.2105/AJPH.2012.300677

Kempen, G. I. J. M, Todd, C. J., Van Haastregt, J. C. M, Rixt Zijlstra, G. A., Beyer, N., Freiberger, E., … Yardley, L. (2007). Cross-cultural validation of the falls efficacy scale international (FES-I) in older people: results from Germany, the Netherlands and the UK were satisfactory. *Disability & Rehabilitation, 29*(2), 155–162. doi: 10.1080/09638280600747637

Kendall-Taylor, N. (2017). *Framing stories for change.* Retrieved from https://climateaccess.org/resource/framing-stories-change.

Kwasnicka, D., Dombrowski, S. U., White, M., & Sniehotta, F. (2016). Theoretical explanations for maintenance of behaviour change: a systematic review of behaviour theories. *Health Psychology Review, 10*(4), 277–296. doi: 10.1080/17437199.2016.115137

Lachman, M. E., Jette, A., Tennstedt, S., Howland, J., Harris, B. A., & Peterson, E. (1997). A cognitive–behavioural model for promoting regular physical activity in older adults. *Psychology, Health & Medicine, 2*(3), 251–261. doi: 10.1080/13548509708400583

Lally, P., & Gardner, B. (2013). Promoting habit formation. *Health Psychology Review, 7*(1), S137–S158. doi: 10.1080/17437199.2011.603640

Lam, P. *Comparing Chen and Sun styles.* www.taichiforhealthinstitute.org/

LeBoff, M. S., Kohlmeier, L., Hurwitz, S., Franklin, J., Wright, J., & Glowacki, J. (1999). Occult vitamin D deficiency in postmenopausal US women with acute hip fracture. *Journal of the American Geriatrics Society, 281*(16), 1505–1511. doi: 10.1001/jama.281.16.1505

Liddle, J. L. M., Lovarini, M., Clemson, L. M., Jang, H. Y., Willis, K., Lord, S. R., & Sherrington, C. (2017). Men's perspectives on fall risk and fall prevention following participation in a group-based programme conducted at Men's Sheds, Australia. *Health & Social Care in the Community, 25*(3), 1118–1126. doi: 10.1111/hsc.12412

Lord, S. R., & Dayhew, J. (2001). Visual risk factors for falls in older people. *Journal of the American Geriatrics Society, 49*(5), 508–515. doi: 10.1046/j.1532-5415.2001.49107.x

Lord, S. R., Smith, S. T., & Menant, J. C. (2010). Vision and falls in older people: risk factors and intervention strategies. *Clinics in Geriatric Medicine, 26*(4), 569–581. doi: 10.1016/j.cger.2010.06.002

Mahoney, J. E. (2015). "Stepping On": stepping over the chasm from research to practice. *Frontiers in Public Health, 2,* 148. doi: 10.3389/fpubh.2014.00148

Mahoney, J., Clemson, L., & Lovarini, M. (2015). Stepping On, a community-based fall prevention program. In M. L. Malone, E. Capezuti, & R. M. Palmer (Eds.), *Geriatrics models of care: bringing 'best practice' to an aging America* (pp. 193–198). Switzerland: Springer International Publishing.

Mahoney, J., Clemson, L., Schlotthauer, A., Mack, K., Shea, T., Gobel, V., & Cech, S. (2017). Modified Delphi consensus to suggest key elements of Stepping On falls prevention program. *Frontiers in Public Health* 2017, *5*(4), 21. doi: 10.3389/fpubh.2017.00021

Mahoney, J. E., Gobel, V. L., Shea, T., Janczewski, J., Cech, S., & Clemson, L. (2016). Improving fidelity of translation of the Stepping On falls prevention program through root cause analysis. *Frontiers in Public Health, 4,* 251. doi: 10.3389/fpubh.2016.00251

Mahoney, J. E., Shea, T. A., Przybelski, R., Jaros, L., Gangnon, R., Cech, S., & Schwalbe, A. (2007). Kenosha County falls prevention study: a randomized, controlled trial of an intermediate-intensity, community-based multifactorial falls intervention. *Journal of the American Geriatrics Society, 55*(4), 489–498. doi: 10.1111/j.1532-5415.2007.01144.x

Mandelbaum, C., Clemson, L., Glassman, M., Williams, R., Silianoff, T., Lipsey, K., & Stark, S. (2019). A scoping review of fall hazards in the homes of older adults and development of a framework for assessment and intervention. Manuscript under review.

Manty, M., Heinonen, A., Viljanen, A., Pajala, S., Koskenvuo, M., Kaprio, J., & Rantanen, T. (2009). Outdoor and indoor falls as predictors of mobility limitation in older women. *Age and Ageing, 38*(6), 757–761. doi:10.1093/ageing/afp178

Mathias, U. S. L., Nayak, B., & Isaacs, B. (1986). Balance in elderly patients: the 'Get Up and Go' test. *Archives of Physical and Medical Rehabilitation*; *67*(6), 387–389.

Mazzeo, R. S., Cavanagh, P., Evans, W. J., Fiatarone, M., Hagberg, J., McAuley, E., & Startzell, J. (1998). The American College of Sports Medicine position stand: exercise and physical activity for older adults. *Medicine & Science in Sports & Exercise, 30*(6), 992–1008.

Menant, J. C., Steele, J. R., Menz, H. B., Munro, B. J., & Lord, S.R. (2009a). Effects of walking surfaces and footwear on temporo–spatial gait parameters in young and older people. *Gait & Posture, 29*(3), 392–7. doi: 10.1016/j.gaitpost

Menant, J. C., Steele, J. R., Menz, H. B., Munro, B. J., & Lord, S. R. (2009b). Rapid gait termination: effects of age, walking surfaces and footwear characteristics. *Gait & Posture, 30*(1), 65–70. doi: 10.1016/j.gaitpost.2009.03.003

Menant, J. C., Steele, J. R., Menz, H. B., Munro, B. J., & Lord, S. R. (2008). Optimizing footwear for older people at risk of falls. *Journal of Rehabilitation Research and Development, 45*(8), 1167–1182. doi: 10.1682/JRRD.2007.10.0168

Menz, H. B., Lord, S. R., & McIntosh, A. S. (2001). Slip resistance of casual footwear: implications for falls in older adults. *Gerontology, 47*(3), 145–149. doi: 10.1159/000052788

Menz, H. B., Morris, M. E., & Lord, S. R. (2006). Foot and ankle risk factors for falls in older people: a prospective study. *Journals of Gerontology – Series A Biological Sciences and Medical Sciences, 61*(8), 866–870. doi:10.1093/gerona/61.8.866

Menz, H. B., Morris, M. E., & Lord, S. R. (2005). Foot and ankle characteristics associated with impaired balance and functional ability in older people. *Journals of Gerontology – Series A Biological Sciences and Medical Sciences, 60*(12), 1546–1552. doi: 10.1093/gerona/60.12.1546

Michie, S., Atkins, L., & West, R. (2014). *The behaviour change wheel: a guide to designing interventions.* Great Britain: Silverback Publishing.

Mickle, K. J., Munro, B. J., Lord, S. R., Menz, H. B., & Steele, J. R. (2010). Foot pain, plantar pressures, and falls in older people: a prospective study. *Journal of the American Geriatrics Society, 58*(10), 1936–1940. doi: 10.1111/j.1532-5415.2010.03061.x

Mickle, K. J., Munro, B. J., Lord, S. R., Menz, H. B., & Steele, J. R. (2009). ISB Clinical Biomechanics Award 2009. Toe weakness and deformity increase the risk of falls in older people. *Clinical Biomechanics, 24*(10), 787–791. doi: 10.1016/j.clinbiomech.2009.08.011

Morin, C. M., Mimeault, V., & Gagne, A. (1999). Nonpharmacological treatment of late-life insomnia. *Journal of Psychosomatic Research, 46*(2), 103–116. doi: 10.1016/S0022-3999(98)00077-4

Nishtala, P. S., Narayan, S. W., Wang, T., & Hilmer, S. N. (2014). Associations of drug burden index with falls, general practitioner visits, and mortality in older people. *Pharmacoepidemiology & Drug Safety, 23*(7), 753–758. doi: 10.1002/pds.3624

Nyman, S. R., Ballinger, C., Phillips, J. E., & Newton, R. (2013). Characteristics of outdoor falls among older people: a qualitative study. *BMC Geriatrics, 13*(1), 125. doi:10.1186/1471-2318-13-125

O'Loughlin, J. L., Robitaille, Y., Boivin, J. F., & Suissa, S. (1993). Incidence of and risk factors for falls and injurious falls among the community-dwelling elderly. *American Journal of Epidemiology, 137*(3), 342–354. doi: 10.1093/oxfordjournals.aje.a116681

Ory, M. G., Smith, M. L., Jiang, L., Lee, R., Chen, S., Wilson, A. D., … Parker, E. M. (2014). Fall prevention in community settings: results from implementing Stepping On in three states. *Frontiers in Public Health, 2*, 232. doi: 10.3389/fpubh.2014

Petch, E., & Smith, E. (1998). *Home safe home road show. Injury prevention for older people in the community.* Toronto, ON: South Riverdale Community Health Centre & Home Safe Committee of Toronto.

Peterson, E. W., & Clemson, L. (2008). Understanding the role of occupational therapy in fall prevention for community dwelling older adults. *OT Practice, 13*(3), CE1–CE7.

Peterson, D. J., Christiansen, A. L., Guse, C. E., & Layde, P. M. (2015). Community translation of fall prevention interventions: the methods and process of a randomized trial. *Journal of Community Psychology, 43*(8), 1005–1018. doi: 10.1002/jcop.21728

Pighills, A., Ballinger, C., Pickering, R., & Chan, S. (2016). A critical review of the effectiveness of environmental assessment and modification in the prevention of falls amongst community dwelling older people. *British Journal of Occupational Therapy, 79*(3): 133–143. doi:10.1177/0308022615600181

Pit, S. W., Byles, J. E., Henry, D. A., Holt, L., Hansen, V., & Bowman, D. A. (2007). A Quality Use of Medicines program for general practitioners and older people: a cluster randomised controlled trial. *The Medical Journal of Australia, 187*(1), 23–30.

Podsiadlo, D., & Richardson, S. (1991). The timed 'Up & Go': a test of basic functional mobility for frail elderly persons. *Journal of the American Geriatrics Society, 39*(2), 142–148. doi: 10.1111/j.1532-5415.1991.tb01616.x

Polkinghorne, D. E. (1988). *Narrative knowing and the human sciences.* Albany, NY: University of New York Press.

Prestwich, A., Lawton, R., & Conner, M. (2003). The use of implementation intentions and the decision balance sheet in promoting exercise behaviour. *Psychology & Health, 18*(6), 707–721. doi:10.1080/0887044031001594493

Ringe, J. D. (2012). The effect of vitamin D on falls and fractures. *Scandinavian Journal of Clinical and Laboratory Investigation, 72*(S243), 73–78. doi: 10.3109/00365513.2012.681965

Robb, S., Burns, D., Docherty, S., & Haase, J. (2011). Ensuring treatment fidelity in a multi-site behavioral intervention study: implementing NIH behavior change consortium recommendations in the SMART Trial. *Psycho-oncology, 20*(11), 1193–1201. doi: 10.1002/pon.1845

Robins, L. M., Hill, K. D., Day, L., Clemson, L., Finch, C., & Haines, T. (2016). Older adult perceptions of participation in group- and home-based falls prevention exercise. *Journal of Aging & Physical Activity, 24*(3), 350–362. doi: 10.1123/japa.2015-0133

Rodriguez, J. C., Dzierzewski, J. M., & Alessi, C. A. (2015). Sleep problems in the elderly. *Medical Clinics of North America, 99*(2), 431–439. doi: 10.1016/j.mcna.2014.11.013

Rosen, T., Mack, K. A., & Noonan, R. K. (2013). Slipping and tripping: fall injuries in adults associated with rugs and carpets. *Journal of Injury and Violence Research, 5*(1), 61–69. doi: 10.5249/jivr.v5i1.177

Rosenkranz, R. R., Kolt, G. S., Brown, J., & Berentson-Shaw, J. (2013). A review of enablers and barriers to physical activity participation among older people of New Zealand and international populations. *International Sports Medicine Journal, 14*(4), 294–312.

Saftari, L. N., & Kwon, O. S. (2018). Ageing vision and falls: a review. *Journal of Physiological Anthropology, 37*(1), 11–14. doi: 10.1186/s40101-018-0170-1

Schlotthauer, A. E., Mahoney, J. E., Christiansen, A. L., Gobel, V. L., Layde, P., Lecey, V., … Clemson, L. (2017). Research on the translation and implementation of Stepping On in three Wisconsin communities. *Frontiers in Public Health, 5*, 128. doi: 10.3389/fpubh.2017.00128

Schneider, B. A., Daneman, M., Murphy, D. R., & Kwong See, S. (2000). Listening to discourse in distracting settings: the effects of ageing. *Psychology & Ageing, 15*(1), 110–125. doi: 10.1037/0882-7974.15.1.110

Sherrington, C., & Menz, H. B. (2003). An evaluation of footwear worn at the time of fall-related hip fracture. *Age & Ageing, 32*(3), 310–314. doi: 10.1093/ageing/32.3.310

Sherrington, C., Michaleff, Z., Fairhall, N., Paul, S., Tiedemann, A., Whitney, J., … Lord, S. R. (2016). Exercise to prevent falls in older adults: an updated systematic review and meta-analysis. *British Journal of Sports Medicine, 51*(24), 1749–1749. doi: 10.1136/bjsports-2016-096547

Sherrington, C., Tiedemann, A., Fairhall, N., Close, J. C. T., & Lord, S. R. (2011). Exercise to prevent falls in older adults: an updated meta-analysis and best practice recommendations. *New South Wales Public Health Bulletin, 22*(3–4), 78–83.

Shumway-Cook, A., & Woollacott, M. H. (2001). *Motor control: theory and practical applications.* Philadelphia, PA: Lippincott, Williams & Wilkins.

Spink, M. J., Menz, H. B., Fotoohabadi, M. R., Wee, E., Landorf, K. B., Hill, K. D., & Lord, S. R. (2011). Effectiveness of a multifaceted podiatry intervention to prevent falls in community dwelling older people with disabling foot pain: randomised controlled trial. *British Medical Journal, 342*(3), d3411–d3411. doi:10.1136/bmj.d3411

Stevens, J. A., Ehrenreich, H., & Mahoney, J. E. (2014). Circumstances and outcomes of falls among high risk community-dwelling older adults. *Gerontologist, 54*, 151.

Strecher, V., McEvoy DeVellis, B., Becker, M., & Rosenstock, I. (1986). The role of self-efficacy in achieving health behaviour change. *Health Education Quarterly, 13*(1), 73–91. doi: 10.1177/109019818601300108

Strommen, J., Brotherson, S., & Yang, Z. (2017). Older adult knowledge and behaviour change in the Stepping On fall prevention program in a community setting. *Journal of Human Sciences & Extension, 5*(3), 99–121.

Tencer, A. F., Koepsell, T. D., Wolf, M. E., Frankenfeld, C. L., Buchner, D. M., Kukull, W. A., … Tautvydas, M. (2004). Biomechanical properties of shoes and risk of falls in older adults. *Journal of the American Geriatrics Society, 52*(11), 1840–1846. doi: 10.1111/j.1532-5415.2004.52507.x

Tiedemann A. (2006). The development of a validated falls risk assessment for use in clinical practice [PhD Thesis]. Sydney, NSW: University of New South Wales. Retrieved from http://unsworks.unsw.edu.au/fapi/datastream/unsworks:1216/SOURCE02

Tinetti, M. E., McAvay, G. J., Fried, T. R., Allore, H. G., Salmon, J. C., Foody, J. M., Bianco, L., Ginter, S., Fraenkel, L. (2008). Health outcome priorities among competing cardiovascular, fall injury, and medication-related symptom outcomes. *Journal of the American Geriatrics Society, 56*, 1409–1416. doi:10.1111/j.1532-5415.2008.01815.x

Tobis, J. S., Reinsch, S., Swanson, J. M., Byrd, M., & Scharf, T. (1985). Visual perception dominance of fallers among community-dwelling older patients. *Journal of American Geriatric Society, 33*(5), 330–333.

Turner, V. (1974). *Dramas, fields, and metaphors: symbolic action in human society.* Ithaca, NY: Cornell University Press.

University of Otago Medical School (2003). *Otago Exercise Program to prevent falls in older adults.* Dunedin NZ: Department of Medicine and Surgical Sciences, University of Otago Medical School.

Vallmuur, K., Eley, R., & Watson, A. (2016). Falls from ladders in Australia: comparing occupational and non-occupational injuries across age groups. *Australian & New Zealand Journal of Public Health, 40*(6):559–563. doi: 10.1111/1753-6405.12592

Vance, E., Delbaere, K., & Lord, S. (2015). Home safety interventions to prevent falls: a mini review. *Falls Links, NSW Fall Prevention Network, 10*(4), 2–6.

van der Velde, N., Stricker, B. H. C., Pols, H. A. P., & van der Cammen, T. J. M. (2007). Risk of falls after withdrawal of fall-risk-increasing drugs: a prospective cohort study. *British Journal of Clinical Pharmacology, 63*(2), 232–237. doi: 10.1111/j.1365-2125.2006.02736.x

Vestibular Disorders Association. (2008). *Figure 1. Balance is achieved and maintained by a complex set of sensorimotor control systems.* http:// vestibular.org/understanding-vestibular-disorder/human-balance-system

Voukelatos, A., Cumming, R. G., Lord, S. R., & Rissel, C. (2007). A randomized, controlled trial of Tai Chi for the prevention of falls: the Central Sydney Tai Chi trial. *Journal of American Geriatric Society, 55*(8), 1185–1191. doi:10.1111/j.1532-5415.2007.01244.x

Waldron, N., Hill, A., & Barker, A. (2012). Falls prevention in older adults. Assessment and management. *Australian Family Physician, 41*(12), 930–935.

Woolcott, J. C., Richardson, K. J., Wiens, M. O., Patel, B., Marin, J., Khan, K. M., & Marra, C. A. (2009). Meta-analysis of the impact of 9 medication classes on falls in elderly persons. *Archives of Internal Medicine, 169*(21), 1952–1960. doi: 10.1001/archinternmed.2009.357

Index